Also by Carl Jones:

Sharing Birth: A Father's Guide to Giving Support during Labor

After the Baby is Born

Mind over Labor

The New Father: Survival Guide (co-author)

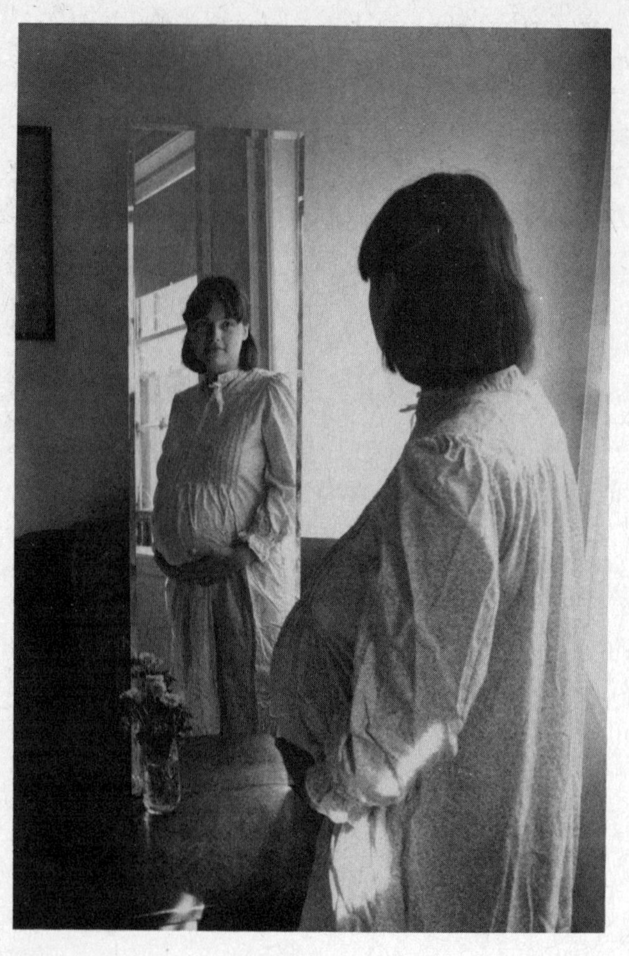

Birth Without Surgery

A Guide to Preventing Unnecessary Cesareans

Carl Jones

Photographs by Jan Sandberg

DODD, MEAD & COMPANY • New York

Published by Dodd, Mead & Company, Inc.
71 Fifth Avenue, New York, N.Y. 10003
Manufactured in the United States of America

1 2 3 4 5 6 7 8 9 10

Library of Congress Cataloging-in-Publication Data

Jones, Carl.
Birth without surgery.

Bibliography: p.
Includes index.
1. Natural childbirth. 2. Cesarean Section—Prevention.
3. Pregnant women—Health and hygiene. I. Title.
RG661.J576 1987 618.4 87–27160
ISBN 0–396–08922–4

Contents

Acknowledgements

My heartfelt thanks to those who have read the manuscript and given me encouragement and suggestions.

To Beth Shearer, the co-founder of C/SEC (Cesareans/ Support, Education and Concern), a childbirth professional who combines profound scholarship with unremitting dedication to helping childbearing parents achieve safe, happy births, my special thanks for providing me with innumerable medical studies, reading the manuscript, and making several changes.

My special thanks to David Stewart, Executive Director of NAPSAC International (The National Association for Parents and Professionals for Safe Alternatives in Childbirth) for offering many fine suggestions.

My gratitude to Don Creevy, M.D., for reading the manuscript and giving valuable suggestions.

Thanks also to Richard Porreco, M.D., for many valuable suggestions. I am also very grateful to Roberta Donahue and Shirley Grainger of Dana Biomedical Library at Dartmouth-Hitchcock Medical Center, Hanover, New Hampshire, both of whom helped me considerably with the research.

Above all, my gratitude to my wife, Jan, who typed the manuscript, and corrected my innumerable errors.

Foreword

What is responsible for the scandalous increase in our cesarean rate?

Is it the trial lawyers? Those who defend us say, "Do more cesareans. If you perform a cesarean you are less likely to lose a suit." Those who press suits against us assert, "The cesarean was performed too late."

Is it our space-age miracle, the electronic fetal monitor? The enthusiasts tell us that routine use is mandatory and there is no value in the simple, traditional stethoscope. However, research articles in respected medical journals state that the use of the fetal monitor has no impact on fetal outcome as compared to one-to-one nursing care with periodic fetal heart auscultation.

Is it because vaginal breech delivery is becoming a lost art, as fewer and fewer residency programs teach the technique? Several generations of otherwise well-trained obstetricians must deliver breech babies by cesarean because they have not learned how to deliver them vaginally. Yet the medical literature is filled with studies claiming vaginal breech delivery to be safe in selected cases.

Is it the reluctance of most obstetricians to attend vaginal deliveries for women with previous cesareans? When the "once a cesarean, always a cesarean" policy is followed, cesareans beget more cesareans. Yet European obstetricians have taken it for granted for many years that a woman having a cesarean will most likely deliver subsequent babies vaginally. And our own medical literature abounds with articles supporting the safety of vaginal birth after cesarean (VBAC), proving that a properly conducted VBAC is actually much safer for mother and perhaps baby than elective repeat cesarean.

All of these factors are to blame for our cesarean rate.

And there is another: Obstetricians are trained in gynecology, a surgical speciality. They are used to performing surgery. Consider the enormous number of hysterectomies, a substantial portion of which many experts believe are performed unnecessarily. Or episiotomies (surgical incisions made to enlarge the birth outlet when the baby is born), which have been called "American obstetrics' gift to the art" despite the fact that there has never been scientific support for their use. Cesarean surgery is yet another of the most widely abused operations.

The fact remains: It has never been and probably never will be proven that a cesarean rate of over 20% is associated with improved fetal outcome as compared to a rate of 3–10%. The maternal mortality rate for cesarean remains at least double that of vaginal delivery, and as much as thirty times greater in some studies. Yet the cesarean rate in the United States continues on its inexorable upward path.

That's why this is an extremely important book. In fact, it is so important that if I had to name three books expectant parents should read, this would be one of them. This concrete, step-by-step guide not only shows how to reduce the fear and pain of normal labor and how to have a better, safer birth. And it works! It should be required reading for all expectant parents. And, I might add, for all physicians.

Don Creevy, M.D.

Birth Without Surgery

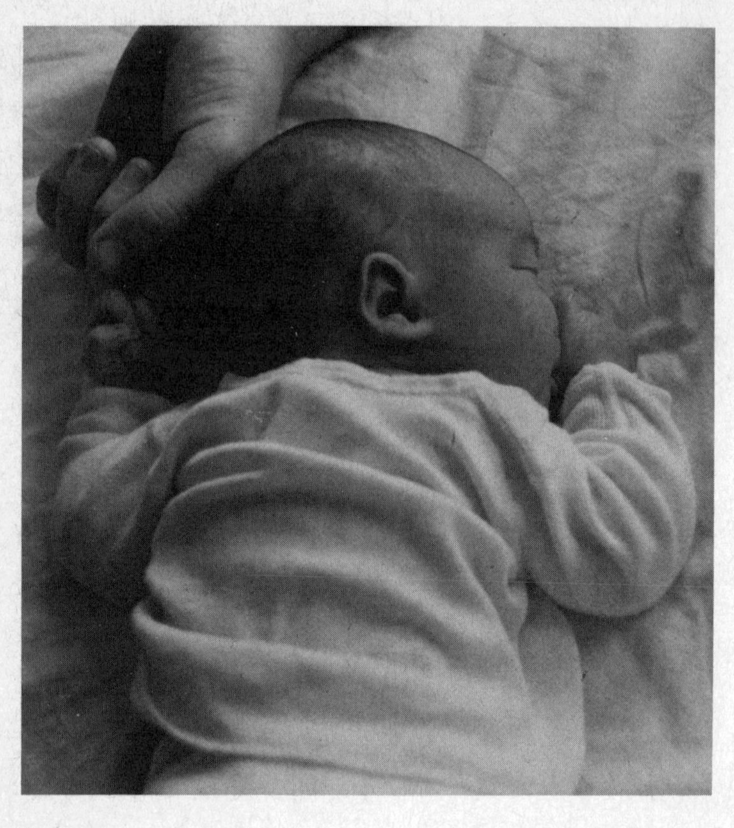

chapter one

Wildfire

Never before in the history of childbirth have expectant parents faced the high risk they do today of birthing surgically. Every pregnant woman faces the possibility. As soon as she enters the hospital in labor, she has a greater than 20 percent chance of being anesthetized, her rolling belly slit open with a sterile scalpel, her baby delivered abdominally—or, as it is euphemistically referred to, "from above." Major abdominal surgery. A cesarean section.

Cesarean birth is like an epidemic. And it is spreading like wildfire. More than one in every five American women delivers "from above." Every year, three-quarters of a million mothers give birth via major abdominal surgery.

Meanwhile, the cesarean mother is transformed from a radiantly healthy woman at the height of her creative power to an invalid undergoing major surgery. Her loss is great. There, on the operating table, she is denied one of life's most precious moments—the supreme thrill of reaching down and touching her baby as it is born, of lifting the child up as it emerges slippery and moist from her body and taking it to her breast. Can anyone wonder why she so often grieves?

Thousands of new parents see their dreams for a happy, normal birth shattered. A cesarean section, usually unexpected, alters their plans for a normal beginning to parenthood. They often leave the hospital frustrated, disappointed, confused, wishing things had been different.

One in every five American women. An incredible thought. Why? The human body has not changed, but American childbirth has. The surgical birth rate has gone out of control. Like wildfire.

In the face of these alarming statistics, the startling fact remains that most of the tremendous number of cesareans in the United States are unnecessary, and most can be prevented.

Almost every woman who can conceive a child can give birth normally and naturally. After all, the body creates from a minute speck a new human being. To meet the needs of the growing and developing baby, a woman's body alters in incredible ways. The placenta, that amazing organ through which passes all of the baby's food and oxygen, is created. The curly bluish umbilical cord is formed. The uterus grows to 500 times its prepregnant capacity. The vagina and cervix soften so that they will open like a blossoming flower on the day of birth. The birth process was designed to work efficiently, beautifully. Women were designed to birth naturally.

Unless there are unusual medical complications, you *can* birth normally, naturally. Nine times out of ten, you *can* prevent cesarean surgery.

This book will show you how.

INCREDIBLE FACTS AND FIGURES

In 1956, a group of Los Angeles physicians were placed on probationary status by the Joint Committee on Accreditation of the American Medical Association and the American Hospital Association because their cesarean rates were almost as high as 10 percent. At that time, the U.S. average was 4 to 5 percent. Today, thirty years later the U.S. average has more than *quadrupled* to 22.7 percent.[1] In some hospitals, the cesarean rate is even higher—30 percent, even 40 percent.[2] Hospitals have actually reported 50 percent cesarean rates. Physicians who now do 10 percent cesareans can boast of a low surgical birth rate (though this is at least triple what a good caregiver's cesarean rate should be).

Occasionally, a cesarean section preserves the health of the mother and/or baby. Under such circumstances, it is warranted, and the intervention is welcome. But this is the exception rather than the rule. I personally believe the cesarean rate should be no higher than 5–6 percent. However, many disagree. In any case, there is no justification for a cesarean rate anywhere near as high as our national average.

Many parents and health professionals believe that the increased surgical birth rate correlates with an improved infant survival rate. This is a myth. A decrease in perinatal mortality rates has somewhat paralleled the increase in the surgical birth rate. However, as Dr. Richard Porreco points out in an article in *Obstetrics and Gynecology,* "The two events are not necessarily causally related."[3] In fact, Iain Chalmers, the well-known epidemiologist, has shown that decreased perinatal mortality can just as well be attributed to the declining stork population in the Netherlands.

Actually, the perinatal mortality rate began improving

years *before* the surge in cesarean deliveries. The improvement is likely the result of better nutrition, better prenatal care, liberalization of abortion, improved neonatal care, *judicious* use of medical intervention, and other factors wholly unrelated to cesarean birth.[4]

In a revealing study conducted at St. Luke's Hospital in Denver, Colorado, Dr. Porreco compared two groups of mothers. In one group, labors were managed with the goal of minimizing the surgical birth rate. The others had no such management. The cesarean rate in the first group was 5.7 percent, compared with a rate of 17.6 percent in the other group. *There were no significant differences in infant outcome,* the Apgar scores* being "virtually identical."[5] Several other studies have clearly demonstrated this.[6,7]

Concerned about the rising cesarean rate, the National Institutes of Health (NIH) organized a conference on cesarean childbirth in 1980. Their task force was made up of professionals in obstetrics, psychology, law, family practice, and sociology, as well as a health-care consumer, to investigate the surgical birth rate. They discovered a startling fact: Our soaring surgical birth rate is paralleled by *no significant improvement in maternal-infant mortality or morbidity.*

"The consensus statement reflects the judgment that this trend of rising cesarean birth rates may be stopped and perhaps reversed while continuing to make improvements in maternal and fetal outcome."[8] At the time of the conference, the cesarean rate was 15.2 percent. It has since risen to 22.7 percent.

* The Apgar score is taken at one and five minutes after birth and evaluates the infant's condition on the basis of heart rate, color, respiration, muscle tone, and reflexes.

One would suspect that the cesarean rate would increase among high-risk pregnancies—mothers with potentially life-threatening complications. This is often not the case, however. According to one study, high-risk centers have a surprisingly *lower* rate than other hospitals.[9]

A single glance at the rising surgical birth rate should be enough to convince anyone that the overwhelming majority of cesarean sections are avoidable. No one needs a battery of medical studies to suggest that a 22.7 percent rate is outrageous. No one should have to be convinced that many, if not most, cesareans are avoidable. No sane person can actually believe that one of every five American women must give birth via major abdominal surgery!

Thanks to consumer pressure and the activity of various cesarean prevention groups, cesarean surgery is now a dominant theme in American childbirth. A cesarean section is something almost every expectant parent wants to avoid. Yet despite the intervention of consumers, concerned physicians, and even the government, the cesarean rate continues to rise.

Cesarean birth has become so widespread—one might even say so popular—that many childbirth professionals and parents have begun to think of it as a normal alternative, simply another way to have a baby. Like lovemaking, vaginal birth is a natural process. Major abdominal surgery, on the other hand, is anything but normal.

One often hears a new mother say, "The cesarean section saved my baby." For that she is grateful. But we must look deeper. Saved her baby from what? In rare cases, surgery has saved the baby from a life-threatening complication. But more often than not, it has deprived the baby and the mother from the benefits of a normal birth.

You have every reason to avoid surgery.

Though the rising surgical birth rate is not paralleled by an improvement in the health of mothers and babies, it is paralleled by an increase in human suffering and gross wastage in terms of economics. Cesarean surgery is not simply another way to have a baby. The cesarean parents have it harder all around.

SURGICAL BIRTH TRAUMA: THE PARENTS' STORY

The scar on the mother's belly is not the only one that follows surgical birth. The cesarean parents suffer from *surgical birth trauma*, a constellation of physical and emotional problems that can effect the entire family.

As Peggy, a cesarean mother and childbirth educator, acknowledged, "No matter how brave and cheerful I decided to be afterwards, it *hurt.* It hurt to move; it hurt to nurse; it hurt to have to ask for help; and it hurt to say I'd had a cesarean birth."[10]

When the otherwise natural event of birth—an experience associated with pride, elation, awe, and joy—is suddenly turned into major abdominal surgery, it can hardly fail to produce trauma. During and after birth, the cesarean family is in a unique position. They suffer burdens not shared by those who birth naturally.

Surgical birth trauma is a four-fold problem, consisting of:

1. the unique physical problems of the cesarean mother;
2. maternal-infant separation and its consequences;
3. the emotional consequences of cesarean birth affecting both parents; and

4. the unique physical problems of the cesarean-born baby.

Physical Trauma

Though mortality among cesarean mothers has dropped considerably over the past few years, Dr. Howard L. Minkoff and Dr. Richard H. Schwartz of Downstate Medical Center in Brooklyn, New York, point out: "When compared to the mortality for women delivered vaginally, the risk of death remains many times higher."[11]

The relative danger of cesarean delivery varies from study to study. According to *Cesarean Childbirth*, the NIH report, cesarean delivery carries two to four times the mortality risk of vaginal birth.[12]

According to the study conducted by Drs. Minkoff and Schwarz, the percentage of mothers with postpartum illness of some sort (endometritis, mastitis, thrombophlebitis, infected wounds, urinary infections, among others) is "10 times greater" among those who have cesarean sections. Among other problems, the cesarean mother incurs the risk of increased chance of hemorrhage with the need for blood transfusion, injury to adjacent organs during the operation, adhesions, aspiration pneumonia, and anesthesia accidents. Though these problems are uncommon, they nevertheless present risks not shared by mothers who birth vaginally.

Meanwhile, the healthy mother must recover from major surgery as well as having given birth. She experiences far greater pain and discomfort than the woman who births naturally. In addition to pain from the stitched incision, the cesarean mother quite frequently suffers postoperative gas pains. While she is learning to deal with the stresses of new motherhood, these discomforts are a major concern.

The trauma to the mother's body, the most obvious consequence of a cesarean, cannot be separated from the emotional burdens surgical childbirth creates. The cesarean mother is less mobile, more dependent on others. This affects her ability to meet her baby's needs, both physically and emotionally. Breastfeeding—just as important to the baby born surgically as it is to the baby born vaginally, if not more so—is more uncomfortable. As a result of this, and perhaps for emotional reasons, cesarean mothers are less likely to breastfeed.

For most new parents, the first few days after birth present difficulties. The transition to parenthood is almost always stressful. Both parents must suddenly become accustomed to their new roles. They must assume the incredible responsibility of being a mother, a father. Their lifestyles are dramatically and irrevocably altered.

For the cesarean parents, this life-altering change is especially difficult. At a time when they must take on a care-providing role, the new mother is in need of care herself. As can be expected, this makes it especially hard for her to adjust to motherhood.

Mothers who have had cesarean births have a more difficult time relating to their infants. The cesarean mother is often more hesitant even to name her baby as a result of interference with the parent-infant attachment process.[13] She is preoccupied with her own feelings, resolving her traumatic birth. Adjusting to motherhood is more difficult since she must first adjust to this experience. Therefore, she is often unable to focus on her infant. This problem is worsened if she has had general anesthesia and was not awake for the birth.

Her hospital stay is prolonged by an average of 3.1 days.[14] If the mother gives birth normally at a childbearing center or hospital, she can return home within twelve to twenty-four hours or less. If she gives birth at home, the traumatic shift to and from an unfamiliar environment during this highly sensitive time is avoided altogether. However, the cesarean mother must remain away from her home from two to seven days, five days being the average.

During the immediate postpartum era, the new mother is emotional, vulnerable, highly sensitive to her environment. Being away from home and separated from her family has a far greater impact than it might have at a less emotionally vulnerable time.

Hospitals may provide the best birthing environment for mothers who have serious medical problems, but a hospital is hardly a conducive setting to begin a new family. Birth is an intimate occasion. The mother who is able to be with her baby, surrounded by family who help her get accustomed to her new role, is far more likely to take new motherhood in stride than the woman in a clinical atmosphere surrounded by strangers.

After a cesarean, there is a far greater burden on the new father. He must (or at least he should) take an additional week from work to be with his partner and baby in the hospital, and later at home. He must take on a greater share of the parenting role, the housekeeping, help his partner get accustomed to breastfeeding, and so forth. In addition, he must give his partner emotional support at a time when he, too, may be frustrated, disappointed, and confused.

Though taking extra time to relate to his infant and be with his wife can help the father make a smoother adjustment to fatherhood, it is far more fulfilling for him to take this time after a vaginal than after a cesarean birth.

Maternal-Infant Separation

Mother and baby are often separated as soon as the baby is delivered. Drs. Marshall Klaus and John Kennel, pioneers in the field of parent-infant attachment, have shown that the first post birth hour is a particularly sensitive time for mothers and babies. This is a time of mutual exploration and *bonding,* that is, developing parent-infant attachment. Of course, bonding can and will take place whether or not mothers and babies are separated during the first few postpartum hours. However, separation is nonetheless emotionally traumatic and interferes with the normal bonding process.

Even if she does remain with her baby, the cesarean mother is denied free expression of her most powerful after-birth instincts—to hold, cuddle, and explore her newborn, bringing her baby immediately to her breast. Someone else, preferably the father, must hold the child for her while she is being stitched.

I suggest in *After the Baby Is Born* that maternal-infant separation may be the major cause of postpartum depression. Throughout her pregnancy, the mother has waited to greet her child. The baby is ready to be taken to the breast immediately following birth. Moreover, nature designed immediate postbirth breastfeeding as a symbiotic process during which baby and mother are mutually benefited. As the baby takes the vitally important colostrum, a premilk secretion rich in nutrients and antibodies that prevent a host of infections, the mother's pituitary gland is stimulated to release the hormone *oxytocin.* Oxytocin causes the uterus to contract, thereby aiding the delivery of the placenta and helping to prevent postpartum hemorrhage. During cesarean surgery, the placenta is delivered via the abdominal incision and the symbiotic process is interrupted.

Emotional Trauma

"There is no comparison between vaginal birth and having a section," said one mother who had experienced a cesarean birth followed by a vaginal birth two years later. "I would never have another cesarean unless my very life depended on it."

Most parents who have had both vaginal and cesarean births emphasize the tremendous difference. Another mother said, "I'd prefer vaginal delivery any day. You feel better so much quicker and there is a state of euphoria that you don't get with a cesarean. And there is something about having a cesarean: it is not *normal.* It is an *abnormal* process and other women look down on you because you had to have one. This baby is so much more sleepy than my last one [born vaginally]."[15]

Whether or not there are those foolish enough to look down on someone who has had a cesarean, many mothers do feel that a cesarean birth carries social stigma. In any case, surgical birth *is* abnormal.

In the main, hospitals have become improved environments for having a baby. A more humanistic, family-centered maternity care is evolving. Mothers and fathers are treated better, and most, but certainly not all, hospitals now welcome the father in the delivery room during a cesarean. Nevertheless, surgical birth has profound psychological consequences. Many parents carry emotional scars for months, even years, after a cesarean.

Parents react differently when the decision to have a cesarean is made. The most common response, of course, is fear.

Many agree to a cesarean only out of exhaustion and despair. The cesarean section often comes as a shock, a terrible disappointment, or, as one mother put it, "something I had never planned for."

Many are relieved that labor is finally over, particularly if it has been long and difficult. A few actually seem unconcerned about how the baby is born and leave the decision entirely in their caregivers' hands, then later regret having had surgery. Many, however, are disappointed from the start. As one would imagine, most cesarean parents are left with a quite negative impression of the birth experience.

As Nicki Royall, author of *You Don't Have to Have a Repeat Cesarean,* and a mother who has experienced both cesarean birth and a vaginal birth after her cesarean, states: "After fifteen hours of unproductive labor, I felt momentary relief when the doctor said I'd need a cesarean. Yet, after the birth of our little girl, Hagen, my emotions changed quickly from a sense of gratitude that we were all right to a sense of loss of femininity. I felt cheated out of one of life's most rewarding experiences, and *guilty.* Somehow, the cesarean was *my fault.* If I'd handled my pregnancy differently, I thought, the outcome might have been different."[16]

Those who have expected and planned for a natural birth are usually the ones to suffer the most. Surgical birth is often a severe blow for which grief is an appropriate reaction. The mother may be angry, particularly if she believes her section was unnecessary. She may feel cheated, deprived of normal birth, abused. Often the mother is justified in such feelings. Many have been cheated. Many have been abused—sometimes by well-meaning health professionals, sometimes by insensitive ones who have cast them in the role of invalids when at the height of their creative power.

Why didn't my body work as a woman's should? is a question many cesarean mothers ask themselves. Giving birth is a part of a woman's sexuality, her self-image. The cesarean mother often feels as though her body has failed her. Many also feel that they have let their husbands down after surgical birth. Frequently, the cesarean mother doesn't know why she feels so sad. She thinks she should be happy that she has a healthy baby, yet wonders why she is so depressed.

Like his partner, the expectant father may also react to a cesarean in a variety of ways. Some are relieved, believing everything is being done to save the child or mother. Frequently, however, fathers are just as frustrated as their partners when the decision to do a cesarean is made. Their dreams, too, are shattered, especially if they have planned the birth with their partners and have been giving support throughout labor. Of course, the father can and should continue to give support through the cesarean section, but it is hardly the same as taking part in vaginal birth.

Most fathers are afraid for their partner's and baby's safety. To many, the cesarean comes as a shock. The father is perhaps massaging his partner's back, giving her emotional encouragement. Then, suddenly, he and his partner are confronted with a decision, perhaps one they never anticipated—the decision to operate.

After the birth, many cesarean fathers are tormented by feelings of failure, guilt, and inadequacy. They blame themselves for not giving adequate labor support. *I should have done more. Where did I fail?* Many feel they were responsible for protecting their vulnerable laboring partners, even though they are virtually powerless in the hospital.

Some fathers who have been denied the right to witness the birth as a result of restrictive hospital policies are justifiably bitter and angry. They often suffer anguish because they were arbitrarily excluded from the birth of their own child. Months after the event, one father began weeping as he recalled missing his son's birth. Another father, quoted in a revealing study, "Unanticipated Cesarean Birth from the Father's Perspective," by Professor Kathryn Antle May and certified childbirth educator Deanna Tomlinson Sollid, R.N., also began to cry when he recalled the nightmare of his wife's cesarean.[17] He had been literally ordered out of the operating room. No one bothered to give him any explanation about his wife's or baby's condition—a not untypical occurrence. In fact, this study showed that seventy percent of the fathers interviewed had complaints about how the hospital staff treated them. There is no excuse whatsoever for denying the father his right to witness the birth of his own child, yet a few hospitals still carry on this heinous practice.

Increased Financial Burden

Cesarean birth is far more costly than vaginal birth. Additional charges are estimated to be at least $1,550 in hospital costs and $250 in physician's fees.[18] This does not reflect additional pediatrician's fees. The father's taking much-needed paternity leave to be with his family and help his wife creates an additional financial loss, as few men are paid for taking an extra week from work after a cesarean. Hiring a postpartum helper or housekeeper if there are no relatives and friends available to help out presents an additional financial burden.

Ironically, relatives and friends often say to the new cesarean mother something such as "You took it the easy way." It is perplexing that anyone could imagine that major abdominal surgery, which leaves a lifelong scar, is somehow easier than normal birth. Such a comment often leaves the parents feeling confused, wondering why they should be so hurt and sad after a cesarean.

The cesarean parents didn't take it the easy way. In every possible way, they have it more difficult than the couple who births naturally.

Many caregivers don't realize just how much emotional trauma the cesarean parents experience. Some, meaning well, tell the mother, "You have a healthy baby and that's the important thing. It doesn't really matter how the baby was born." Having a healthy baby is the purpose of pregnancy and the end result of pregnancy's climax in labor. However, implying that it doesn't really matter how the baby is born is like saying it doesn't matter how the seed gets in the uterus as long as the egg is fertilized. As Colleen, a cesarean mother, said, "I was not supposed to dwell on the mode of delivery, just on the baby. My disappointment and bitterness deepened as I tried to repress my feelings."[19]

To most parents, how the baby is born *does* matter. Most care whether they birth vaginally or surgically.

SURGICAL BIRTH TRAUMA: THE BABY'S STORY

Some imagine the cesarean-born baby suffers less birth trauma and has an easier beginning in life than the baby born vaginally. However, like the cesarean mother, the baby has a far more difficult time adjusting.

Judging by appearances, babies born surgically may look neater, more symmetrical. Their skull bones have not molded, that is, adapted to the pelvis during the second stage of labor. After a normal birth, the head looks cone-shaped, pushed in on one side, or somehow lopsided.

However, this is only a temporary condition. The baby's head assumes a normal-looking shape shortly after birth. The skull bones are designed to mold, just as babies are designed to begin extrauterine life after a normal labor and birth.

Despite the neater appearance, babies delivered by cesarean surgery frequently score lower on tests of sucking behavior, neurological response, sensory responses, motor activities, and overall alertness than do babies born vaginally. The cesarean-delivered baby is also at increased risk of jaundice, and, of course, may suffer the effects of anesthesia and other medications used.[20]

Cesarean-delivered babies are far more likely to have breathing difficulties than babies born vaginally. Several studies have shown that an elective repeat cesarean carries an increased risk of delivering a premature infant likely to suffer from *respiratory distress syndrome* (RDS).[21, 22, 23] With RDS, the lungs are unable to function properly, a potentially life-threatening complication. One study showed that even infants who are not mistakenly delivered prematurely are at higher risk of RDS. This study concludes: "It is likely that the respiratory distress in these infants is secondary to the mode of delivery, not the delivery of a premature infant."[24]

Normal labor is healthy stress. Far from being traumatic, labor actually prepares the baby for her first breath. Labor contractions massage the baby and get her ready to make the transition to life outside the womb. They prepare her lungs for the moment when she will be breathing on her own rather than taking oxygen from the blood via the placenta. Fluid is expelled from the lungs during the archetypal rite of passage—the awesome journey through the birth canal.

Adrenaline and noradrenaline, fetal stress hormones produced by the adrenal glands, are released in great quantity in the course of normal labor. These stress hormones, so called because in an older child or adult they trigger the "flight-or-fight" response, belong in a class of biochemicals called catecholamines. During a vaginal delivery, catecholamine levels surge in response to labor contractions, which intermittently deprive the baby of oxygen and later squeeze the baby's head in the birth canal. High catecholamine levels are believed to enhance the baby's ability to function effectively when first separated from the mother.[25]

According to Hugo Lagercrantz and Theodore A. Slotkin, the "resulting surge of hormones prepares the infant to survive outside the womb. It clears the lungs and changes their physiological characteristics to promote normal breathing, mobilizes readily usable fuel to nourish cells, insures that a rich supply of blood goes to the heart and brain and may even promote attachment between mother and child."[26]

Elevated catecholamines also protect the infant from oxygen loss while she is making her dramatic rite of passage. In addition, high levels of catecholamines probably contribute to the infant's alert state the first hour or so following birth. This in turn facilitates the parent-infant attachment process (bonding) during this highly sensitive time.

Unlike the vaginal baby, infants delivered by elective cesarean section without labor have low catecholamine levels. This is perhaps the reason cesarean-born infants frequently have breathing problems. Several studies have shown that the lungs' ability to stretch and efficiently exchange carbon dioxide and oxygen is greater in infants delivered vaginally than among infants delivered by cesarean section.

Clearly it is not only the parents who care whether or not they birth vaginally. It is also important to the baby.

PREVENTION: BETTER THAN RECOVERY

No couple living in America, with its phenomenal 22.7 percent surgical birth rate, can afford to overlook cesarean prevention. Oddly, medical organizations do not yet have any means of regulating cesarean section rates. Therefore, it is up to the parents. You alone must prevent unnecessary surgery. Every expectant parent—whether planning a home, childbearing-center, or hospital birth—should take steps to reduce the likelihood of surgery. Doing so now, during pregnancy, and later during labor, is your only insurance of avoiding surgical birth trauma.

In a very few cases, cesarean surgery is a life-saving operation. The indications for which a cesarean is justified are discussed in the next chapter. Under these unusual circumstances, it makes sense for the mother to recuperate from both birth and major abdominal surgery. Both parents must then accept their rocky beginning to parenthood with the thought that their cesarean was the best choice available.

But in the majority of cases, cesarean surgery does not make sense. It is not justified. Often a cesarean section creeps up insidiously. Without warning, the parents suddenly discover it's too late to do anything. Mother, father, and baby soon find themselves recovering from surgical birth trauma.

You can avoid this unnecessary emotional and physical suffering. Unless there are unusual medical complications, every woman can give birth without surgery. All it takes is an open mind, the desire to birth normally, and the willingness, time, energy, and commitment to follow the steps outlined ahead.

In the following chapters, you will discover what conditions often lead to unnecessary cesarean surgery and what you can do to minimize your chance of surgical birth.

Needless to say, reading this book cannot guarantee birth without surgery. As already stated, surgical delivery is warranted in certain unusual cases. However, if you follow *all* of the steps in the following chapters, you will increase your ability to birth normally, whether or not you have had a previous cesarean.

In addition, if you are among the few who have a necessary cesarean, taking the steps ahead will still prove helpful. They will minimize the effects of surgical birth trauma and make a necessary cesarean as rewarding an experience as possible. If you take preventive steps during pregnancy and labor and still have a cesarean section, at least you will know you have done everything in your power to prevent surgical intervention. Then there will be no cause for self-blame or for feeling as if you should have done things differently. This is a long step toward lessening the negative feelings that so often follow surgical birth.

Meanwhile, bear in mind that truly necessary cesareans are rare. You were designed to birth naturally. Like your wedding, giving birth is one of the truly big occasions in your life. As you take the commonsense steps this guide offers, expect your birth to be a richly rewarding experience—an event never to be forgotten. You, your partner, and your baby deserve it.

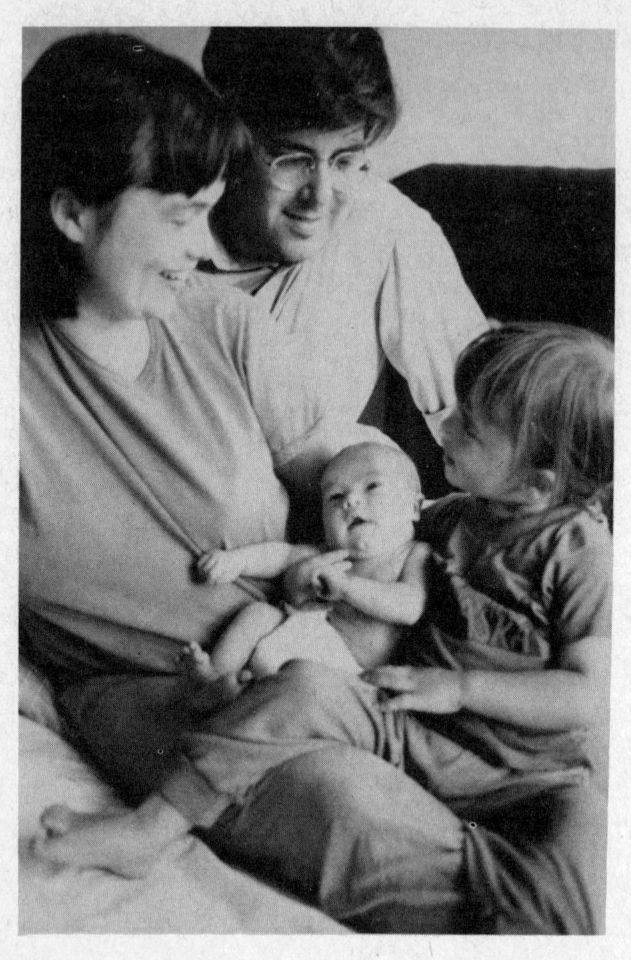

chapter two

The Genuine and the Alleged: Indications for Cesarean Surgery

In October 1984, a woman who was laboring in a Boston hospital began having irregular contractions, a not uncommon occurrence. Her physician suspected cephalopelvic disproportion (CPD), a condition in which the baby's head is supposedly too large to fit through its mother's pelvis. Alleged CPD is one of the prime indications for cesarean surgery in the United States. The physician ordered X-rays to confirm his suspicion. When the X-ray results came back, they did indeed show CPD. The head simply could not fit through the pelvis. The mother would have to have a cesarean.

But it was too late. By the time the X-ray results had come back, the mother had already given birth to a healthy baby *vaginally.*

The few genuine complications prompting a necessary cesarean section have not altered over the past few decades. Yet the mother's risk of surgical delivery has risen dramatically. Why? One reason is that the alleged indications for cesarean birth have changed. CPD is one of the many reasons given for cesarean surgery discussed ahead that is not necessarily valid.

To prevent unnecessary surgery, it is important for the expectant parents to be aware of the difference between genuine and alleged reasons for cesarean delivery.

THE GENUINE

There are rare circumstances in which cesarean delivery is considered necessary, often making a cesarean preferable to vaginal birth.

All of these are rather uncommon problems. The likelihood of some (such as *abruptio placentae* and *preeclampsia/eclampsia*) can be reduced by observing the commonsense rules of good prenatal health such as good nutrition.

Problems such as *fetal distress, pelvic contraction* (a rare condition in which the baby can't fit through the pelvic structure), and *dysfunctional labor* (lack of cervical dilation) all warrant cesarean birth in rare circumstances. However, they are discussed in the next section (on "alleged" reasons for a cesarean) because more often than not they can be corrected without resorting to surgery.

Meanwhile, it is important to remember that many of the following "genuine" conditions *do not always* require surgery.

Placental Abruption (Abruptio Placentae)

All or part of the placenta separates from the uterine wall in this rare condition. Placental abruption occurs most frequently during the third trimester, and sometimes it occurs during labor. It may result in maternal hemorrhaging and fetal distress requiring immediate medical care. A cesarean section is performed to prevent severe bleeding. The baby may still be born healthy as long as the condition is not too severe.

Warning signs of placental abruption are abdominal pain, abdominal tenderness, rigidity of the uterus, and vaginal bleeding (the latter is not always present, as blood sometimes collects under the placenta rather than escaping).

The cause of this condition is unknown, but the problem is often associated with malnutrition and high blood pressure. Good nutrition, therefore, decreases your likelihood of this unusual problem. Very rarely, the placenta separates as a result of a fall or an extremely hard blow to the abdomen. However, falling during pregnancy usually does not affect the baby or uterus.

Placenta Previa

In this rare complication, the placenta covers part or all of the cervix at the time of birth.

The warning sign is painless bleeding late in pregnancy. This occurs as the cervix softens and stretches and part of the placenta detaches. Ultrasound testing will confirm the initial diagnosis. Blood loss is sometimes sufficiently severe to require a transfusion.

If placenta previa is *complete* and the mother is bleeding profusely, the baby should be delivered surgically to prevent severe maternal blood loss and fetal death. If placenta previa is detected before bleeding begins, the cesarean is often done early (at about thirty-eight weeks) following testing for fetal maturity.

A second trimester ultrasound may reveal a low-lying placenta. However, many of these correct themselves before term. The diagnosis should be confirmed in the third trimester.

Normal delivery is frequently possible in the face of *partial* placenta previa, as the pressure of the baby's head often prevents bleeding. In this case, the mother should be carefully observed through labor.

Note that a small amount of vaginal bleeding is usually nothing to be alarmed about. It may follow intercourse or an internal exam as a result of small capillaries breaking in the delicate cervix. However, any vaginal bleeding should be mentioned to your caregiver without delay.

Prolapsed Cord

In this rare condition, the umbilical cord comes through the birth canal in advance of the baby. Prolapsed cord is more common when the baby is in a breech or transverse position or the presenting part is not fully engaged.

When the cord prolapses, it is compressed as the baby descends, cutting off his oxygen supply. A cesarean is performed to prevent the baby's brain damage or death from asphyxia.

Malpresentation

This includes breech presentation and transverse lie. Since a baby in the breech position can frequently be born vaginally, this will be discussed later.

In the transverse lie, the shoulder may present first and the baby most often cannot be delivered vaginally. The most common causes of transverse lie are extreme abdominal laxity (sometimes associated with having had many babies), placenta previa, and true pelvic contraction (the pelvis is too small for the baby).

Herpes

Though herpes is not a very serious disease for the mother, it is often grave for the baby. If the baby is affected, the disease can leave permanent damage or be fatal. The infection is fatal greater than 50 percent of the time.

If the mother has primary (first-time) genital herpes at term, the risk that the newborn will be infected is 40 to 60 percent.[2] If, on the other hand, the mother has a recurrent outbreak, the risk that the baby will be infected is much lower, about 5 percent, according to Alice A. Robinson of the Herpes Resource Center in Palo Alto, California.[3] The risk of infection increases rapidly once the membranes have ruptured.

Fortunately, neonatal herpes is rare. However, every precaution should be taken to prevent the disease. If the mother has active genital lesions, a cesarean is performed shortly after labor begins, and before or as soon as possible after fetal membranes have ruptured.

If you or your partner (or a past sexual partner) has or has had genital herpes, let your caregiver know so potential problems can be ruled out or avoided. An outbreak during pregnancy will usually not affect the baby, and vaginal delivery may still be possible if there is no virus present near the time of birth. However, if the virus is present, the baby could be at risk even in the absence of maternal symptoms.

Generally speaking, if you have a history of herpes, your caregiver will take viral cultures and/or Pap smears beginning at the thirty-second week after your last menstrual period, and repeat the procedures until birth to determine whether or not the virus is present at the time of labor.

Meanwhile, avoid undue stress, eat a well-balanced diet, and get plenty of rest. This decreases your likelihood of a fresh outbreak.

If you have an outbreak near the time of your due date, you may be able to get it to subside by using a variety of therapeutic treatments. The pamphlet "Herpes" includes herbal treatments, acupuncture, and other valuable information. (See Resources.)

Diabetes Mellitus

There is a higher risk of fetal death during the last few weeks of pregnancy with diabetic mothers. Accordingly, a preterm cesarean birth is often done, especially if the condition is severe.

Recently, maternal-infant outcome in the presence of diabetes has improved. This is largely the result of careful management and proper diet during the prenatal months. If the mother's blood sugar is carefully controlled with strict attention to nutrition and periodic insulin injections, she may be able to give birth normally. However, to avoid a cesarean it is essential to find a caregiver who is both an expert with this particular problem and who is willing to help you have a vaginal birth.

Other Maternal Illnesses

A few illnesses contribute to serious complications for either mother or baby and merit cesarean surgery. These include preeclampsia/eclampsia (a disease of pregnancy characterized by hypertension, swelling, and protein in the urine), chronic hypertension, and certain cardiac and kidney diseases.

The baby must often be delivered prematurely to protect either infant or mother. However, frequently an attempt can be made to induce labor before resorting to surgery.

A cesarean is not inevitable just because you have one of the above diseases. Many mothers can still give birth vaginally. It all depends on the individual situation. Be sure to choose a caregiver who fully supports natural birth and who will resort to surgery only if necessary.

THE ALLEGED

As striking as it may seem, *most* of the conditions for which American mothers have cesareans are either not always valid indications for surgery or are avoidable. Obviously a life-threatening problem like abruptio placentae or prolapsed cord may be an emergency requiring immediate medical intervention. However, the problems discussed in this section are by no means as cut and dried.

Many of the following complications, such as genuine fetal distress, certainly justify a cesarean. However, such problems are sometimes created by the medical management of labor and are often avoidable.

Frequently, a so-called indication for cesarean surgery such as failure to progress in labor or CPD can be overcome by other methods far less radical than a cesarean section.

You can decrease your likelihood of most of the problems discussed ahead by following *all* of the steps in Chapters Four and Five.

Changing Conditions and the Rising Cesarean Rate

The rising cesarean rate largely reflects a changing view toward complications of childbirth. Today, more and more complications are becoming acceptable reasons for cesarean surgery.

For example, most obstetricians now deem the breech position, in which the baby's buttocks or feet, rather than his head, present first in the birth outlet (discussed in more detail below), a justifiable reason for a cesarean. Accordingly, 76 percent of all breech babies were born by cesarean in 1983.[4] This represents a radical departure from just thirteen years before, when the cesarean rate for the breech position was 11.6 percent.[5]

According to *Cesarean Childbirth,*[6] 80 to 90 percent of the rise in the U.S. cesarean rate from 1970 to 1978 is the result of four conditions:

- Dystocia (impaired labor, including cephalopelvic disproportion, abnormal maternal pelvis, and prolonged labor)
- Repeat cesarean
- Breech presentation
- Fetal distress

Indication	% of All Cesareans Done for This Indication (1978)	% Contribution to Rise in Rate
Dystocia	31%	30%
Repeat cesarean	31%	25–30%
Breech presentation	12%	10–15%
Fetal distress	5%	10–15%

From *Cesarean Childbirth,* U.S. Department of Health and Human Services, Public Health Service, National Institutes of Health, NIH Publication No. 82-2065, October 1981. Bethesda, MD

Physicians have developed a more liberal attitude toward cesarean surgery. Fifty years ago, a cesarean was performed only for grave emergencies, and the cesarean rate was about 1 percent. Today, however, with advances in anesthesiology and surgical medicine, the operation has become increasingly safe, though it still poses a far higher risk to mother and baby than vaginal birth. It is therefore easier for the physician to make a decision to perform a cesarean.

In some ways, the use of cesarean surgery has improved the outcome for mother and baby. For example, cesarean delivery has largely replaced the use of mid-forceps (application of forceps when the baby's head is high in the pelvis but engaged) because it is often the safer alternative. However, more often than not, cesareans can be avoided in the presence of all the indications described ahead.

Dystocia

Dystocia (from the Greek *dys,* "abnormal," and *tokos,* "childbirth") refers to abnormal labor. However, it actually includes several separate conditions.

All of the following are lumped together under the somewhat vague category of "dystocia": CPD; fetal malpresentation, including the breech position; unusual anomalies of the bones or soft tissues of the maternal pelvis; failure to progress in labor; prolonged labor; uterine inertia; and inefficient uterine contractions.

These are not always entirely separate problems. For instance, CPD is often thought to be the cause of failure of labor to progress. Likewise, fetal malpresentation is frequently at the root of a prolonged labor.

Cephalopelvic Disproportion (CPD)

CPD, or cephalopelvic disproportion, is a condition in which the baby's head is assumed to be too large for the mother's pelvis. Responsible for a tremendous number of cesareans each year, it is one of the most common forms of so-called "dystocia" and is often cited as the reason for failure of labor to progress.

On the surface, CPD might seem like a good reason to deliver a baby surgically. After all, what else can one do if the baby's head is too large to fit through the pelvis? However, the diagnosis of CPD is questionable at best. It is almost impossible to determine if the baby's head is really too large. As Dr. Walter J. Hannah of Women's College Hospital in Toronto points out: "Most feto-pelvic disproportion is relative and often easily overcome by a good labor."[7]

Relative disproportion is often the result of a somewhat small pelvis, a larger-than-average baby, or the baby in a posterior position (bony skull against the spine) or with the chin not well-flexed onto the neck. Overcoming such disproportion is often just a matter of time.

Nature designed both the baby's head and the mother's pelvis to adapt to one another marvelously. Baby and mother prepare to accommodate one another during the latter weeks of pregnancy. At this time, the hormone *relaxin*, produced by the ovaries, is believed to soften the pelvic ligaments (tough connective tissues that hold bones together) as well as the cervix. This ligament softening—responsible for the waddling gait often seen in expectant mothers near term—prepares the otherwise rigid pelvis, which is made up of several bones connected by ligaments, to yield during the birth process and make room for the baby.

During second-stage labor, as the baby is pushed down the birth canal on his miraculous journey to mother's waiting arms, the infant's still-soft skull molds. In other words, the skull adapts to fit the maternal pelvis. Molding is responsible for the sometimes peculiar-shaped heads of newborns. Babies are often born with "cone heads," or skulls that look pushed in on one side. However, they invariably adopt a normal-looking appearance within a few days.

As a result of both pelvic yielding and the molding of the infant's head, the mother can usually give birth vaginally, even if the baby's head is "too large" for her pelvis. X-ray studies have clearly demonstrated the "moldability" of the pelvis during childbearing.[8]

Even if you have a small pelvis, your chances of birthing normally are still good. Many mothers who have been told they have a so-called "inadequate" pelvis can and do birth vaginally.[9] Many who have had cesarean sections for CPD later deliver larger second or third babies vaginally. (This is discussed further in Chapter Six.)

If the baby is large or labor is slow, assuming an upright birth position is often the solution. Squatting, as discussed in Chapter Five, can increase the size of the pelvic outlet an average of 28 percent over the supine (flat on the back) position. Other aids to a prolonged labor (which might result with a large baby) are discussed in Chapter Five.

A few physicians believe they can predict whether or not the mother will require a cesarean by measuring the mother's pelvis and the size of the baby's head via X-ray or ultrasound. However, the story introducing this chapter suggests that even X-ray diagnosis of CPD is wholly unreliable. Several studies have clearly shown that X-rays cannot determine if the baby will fit through the pelvis. In fact, pelvimetry (measuring the pelvis) can probably diagnose only a genuine abnormality, which is considerably uncommon.

True CPD is very rare and can *only* be detected during labor and *after* a period of strong contractions.

Failure to Progress

Failure to progress in labor is the primary indication for cesarean surgery in the United States.[10] Though a cesarean may at times be warranted when labor is dysfunctional or the cervix doesn't dilate, in most cases surgery can be avoided.

Often the problem is nonexistent. Many obstetricians today think in terms of averages when it comes to labor's length and the speed of cervical dilation. As the NIH report points out: "The concept that slow progress constitutes abnormal progress permeates current obstetric thinking."[11] As a result, many physicians and hospitals have a policy of delivering all laboring mothers within twenty-four hours and intervening after two to four hours if there has been poor progress in active labor.

Nature does not always conform to averages. The length of labor varies tremendously from mother to mother. Accordingly, it is sometimes difficult to make a distinction between a labor that has truly failed to progress and one that is simply "resting." Sometimes, labor stops part way through for a while. This doesn't mean the mother should be whisked off to the operating room. Labor often resumes.

Sometimes labor is slow to begin. The mother has a prolonged *prodromal* period that is like an introductory phase of labor. Contractions may occur on and off for several hours or days before the cervix really starts to dilate. *Latent* or *early* labor (dilation to four centimeters) can also go on for a long period before labor becomes active.

According to Dr. Luella Klein, past president of the American College of Obstetricians and Gynecologists and professor at Emory University School of Medicine in Atlanta, Georgia, "Recognition and correct management of prodromal labor and the latent phase of labor should lead to decrease in diagnosis of 'failure to progress' and the impression of a 'prolonged labor.' "[12]

Once labor has become active, slow progress can be the result of lack of fluids, exhaustion, remaining in one position, and the injudicious use of obstetrical medication. Frequently, it results from anxiety. High levels of stress hormones interfere with labor, producing less efficient uterine contractions and a longer first-stage labor.[13]

You can significantly reduce your chance of failure to progress by following the steps in Chapters Four and Five. However, if the problem does occur, you can try many things to get labor going before resorting to medical intervention and surgical birth. This is discussed further in Chapter Five in the section "If Labor Stops or Slows Down."

Repeat Cesarean

Most American mothers who have had cesarean sections deliver subsequent babies by repeat cesarean. However, the vast majority of repeat cesareans are avoidable. Unless there are problems with the *present* pregnancy or the cesarean was for an undoubtedly recurrent cause such as an absolutely contracted pelvis that will not permit the delivery of a normal size baby (a very rare condition that does not include CPD), vaginal birth is almost always the better choice.

Vaginal birth after a previous cesarean is discussed in detail in Chapter Six.

Breech Presentation

In the breech position, the buttocks or feet present first in the birth outlet, rather than the head. The caregiver can let you know if the baby is breech at a prenatal appointment. There are three basic types of breech presentation.

Frank breech—the thighs are flexed and legs folded over the front of the body so the feet touch the head. This is the most favorable for vaginal birth;

Full (*or complete*) *breech*—the legs are crossed on the abdomen (baby sits Indian-style, buttocks and feet presenting to the birth canal first); and

Footling breech—one or both feet present first. This position is associated with a higher risk of prolapsed cord.

Today, most obstetricians deliver all breech babies via cesarean section. As stated earlier, the proportion of breech babies delivered surgically rose sharply from 11.6 percent in 1970 to 80.4 percent in 1985.[14]

Cesarean surgery for breech is self-perpetuating. The more breech babies that are delivered surgically, the less experience residents have in handling vaginal breech births. Accordingly, experts in vaginal breech delivery are becoming less common. The mother who wants a vaginal breech birth may have to look especially hard for a competent caregiver who can fulfill her need.

Several complications are associated with breech babies *regardless* of the mode of delivery. These include birth defects, placenta previa, prolapsed cord, *polyhydramnios* (excessive amniotic fluid) and uterine tumors and other malformations.

Complications can also be associated with vaginal breech birth, including: asphyxia, which can occur if the body passes through the birth canal leaving the head (the largest part) trapped; prolapsed cord; aspiration of fluid during the birth process; and birth injury. Infant mortality is therefore higher with vaginal breech than with vertex, or normal delivery (head down).

Cesarean surgery is often the safest way to deliver the

breech baby. For example, according to the NIH report *Cesarean Childbirth,* the baby presenting as a complete or footling breech, the baby with marked *hyperextension* of the head (chin up rather than well flexed on the chest), and the large baby will have a better outcome if delivered surgically.[15]

However, under the following conditions, the NIH report states, vaginal breech birth should "remain an acceptable obstetrical choice":

1. the baby's anticipated weight is less than eight pounds;
2. the mother has a normal-sized and -shaped pelvis;
3. the baby is in the frank breech position without hyperextended head; and
4. the delivery is conducted by a physician experienced in vaginal breech delivery.[16]

A similar Canadian report acknowledged that cesarean delivery of breech babies was becoming widespread in Canada despite the fact that extensive review of the literature failed to "uncover any evidence to support this trend." The report concludes that cesarean section is not indicated merely because a baby is in the breech position. "Cesarean section should not be performed for breech presentation unless it can be shown to be justified."[17] The report recommends vaginal birth for frank or complete breech at thirty-six weeks or more gestation when the estimated birth weight is 2,500 to 4,000 grams (5.5 to 8.8 pounds) and suggests that vaginal birth be offered as an alternative if the frank or complete breech baby at thirty-one to thirty-five weeks gestation weighs from 1,500 to 2,500 grams (3.5 to 5.5 pounds).[18]

Under the conditions outlined in the Canadian and United States NIH reports, vaginal breech birth is often as safe (if not safer) than cesarean delivery. Another study concludes that "The subsequent health and development of children is similar whether the infant in the breech position is delivered vaginally or by cesarean section."[19] Several studies agree that under proper conditions, vaginal birth is the best route for the breech baby.[20, 21, 22] However, it is essential that you have a caregiver supportive of vaginal breech who can evaluate your particular situation.

Dr. Leo Sorger of Malden, Massachusetts, an expert in breech birth, reminds clients that it is better to have a cesarean than a poorly done vaginal breech. He stresses the importance of choosing a physician or midwife experienced in vaginal breech births. Many midwives are far more experienced in handling vaginal breech than most obstetricians.

Dr. Sorger also recommends that mothers birthing a breech vaginally use an upright position (squatting, standing) as this facilitates delivery.

The mother who plans a vaginal breech birth should be prepared for the possibility of a cesarean on the off chance that labor does not go well—or if the baby remains high in the pelvis (indicating that it may have difficulty fitting through the birth outlet).

Meanwhile, in the majority of cases, the breech baby can be safely turned to a head-first position during the final weeks of pregnancy, thus resolving the cesarean question.

If Your Baby Is in the Breech Position

Until after the thirtieth week, the baby's position doesn't make much difference. Breech babies often turn spontaneously. However, if your baby remains breech after the thirtieth week, there are several ways to turn it to vertex (head down). Consult your caregiver before trying any of the following.

Exercise for turning a breech baby Many have found the following exercise quite effective. According to Dr. Juliet M. DeSouza, it has proven 88.9 percent successful in turning breech babies.[23] Begin doing it around the thirtieth week after your last menstrual period.

> Lie flat on back with knees bent, feet flat on the floor, and pillows or cushions under the buttocks so that the pelvis is nine to twelve inches from the floor.
>
> Assume this position for ten minutes twice daily until the baby turns head down, which often occurs within two to three weeks.

Suzanna May Hilbers, a registered physical therapist and teacher trainer for ASPO/Lamaze, suggests accompanying this exercise with mental imagery. She advises imagining children doing somersaults, clothes tumbling in the dryer, or whatever else gives you a clear image of turning.

External version If the above exercise does not cause the baby to turn, *external version,* that is, turning the breech manually, often works. With hands on the abdomen, the caregiver gently manipulates the baby into the vertex position. This is usually done at thirty to thirty-six weeks after the last menstrual period, and sometimes at the beginning of labor.

External version is usually quite successful in turning a breech. According to Dr. Edward J. Quilligan, external version could "cut the section rate for breech presentation in half."[24] This more than justifies widespread acceptance for the procedure. Oddly, however, few physicians practice external version.

A study by Dr. Brook Ranney shows a 90 percent success

rate with external version.[25] However, many of the babies in this study would probably have turned spontaneously. Dr. Leo Sorger (who usually asks the father to help him turn the breech under his expert guidance) has a 60 to 71 percent success rate. Dr. Thomas J. Garite of Long Beach, California, has a 65 percent success rate.

According to Dr. Garite, contraindications include:

> previous cesarean, placenta previa or third trimester bleeding, premature rupture of membranes or other cause of too little amniotic fluid, uterine malformations, intrauterine growth retardation with signs of fetal distress, cephalopelvic disproportion, or maternal illness such as diabetes or heart disease which could contraindicate the use of tocolytic drugs (agents which relax the uterus).[26]

Rare complications associated with external version include placental abruption and premature birth. Therefore, the procedure is for expert hands only.

If your caregiver doesn't do external version (many are not skilled at this procedure), consult another caregiver who does.

Finally, if turning the breech fails in the physician's or midwife's office, it can be tried in the hospital with a drug to relax the uterus such as Terbutaline Sulfate or Ritodrine.

Acupuncture Acupuncture or *moxibustion* (application of heat to an acupuncture point with an herbal stick called moxa) is frequently quite successful for turning breech babies. According to one study from the People's Republic of China, moxibustion was successful in turning breech babies 90.3 percent of the time.[27] However, like external version, this is to be done by skilled hands only. Consult a licensed acupuncturist for more information.

Fetal Distress

Fetal distress occurs when the baby receives insufficient oxygen. Prolonged fetal distress may lead to brain damage or death and is therefore certainly a valid indication for surgical birth. However, the problem is often avoidable or correctible without surgery.

The best therapy is prevention. Fetal distress frequently results when the mother remains in the supine (flat on the back) position during labor; from epidural anesthesia, which often lowers the mother's blood pressure, causing fetal distress; from the use of Pitocin to augment labor; and from prolonged breath-holding during second-stage contractions. The mother should therefore avoid these causative factors whenever possible.

Fetal distress can also result from maternal anxiety. This can be relieved by choosing a birthing environment conducive to normal labor (discussed in Chapter Four) and having effective labor support (see Chapter Five).

When fetal distress does occur, it can often be corrected with a change of position and by giving the mother oxygen. According to the NIH report, "Operative intervention for fetal distress can be justified when all avenues of correction have been explored and found not to be effective."[28]

Since fetal distress is accompanied by *acidosis* (increased acidity in the fetal blood), many physicians recommend sampling fetal scalp blood to confirm (or rule out) a diagnosis made by reading EFM (electronic fetal monitoring) tracings before resorting to surgical delivery. Fetal scalp blood pH sampling has been found to lower the incidence of cesarean surgery in the presence of suspected fetal distress. (This procedure is described in the section on electronic fetal monitoring in Chapter Three.)

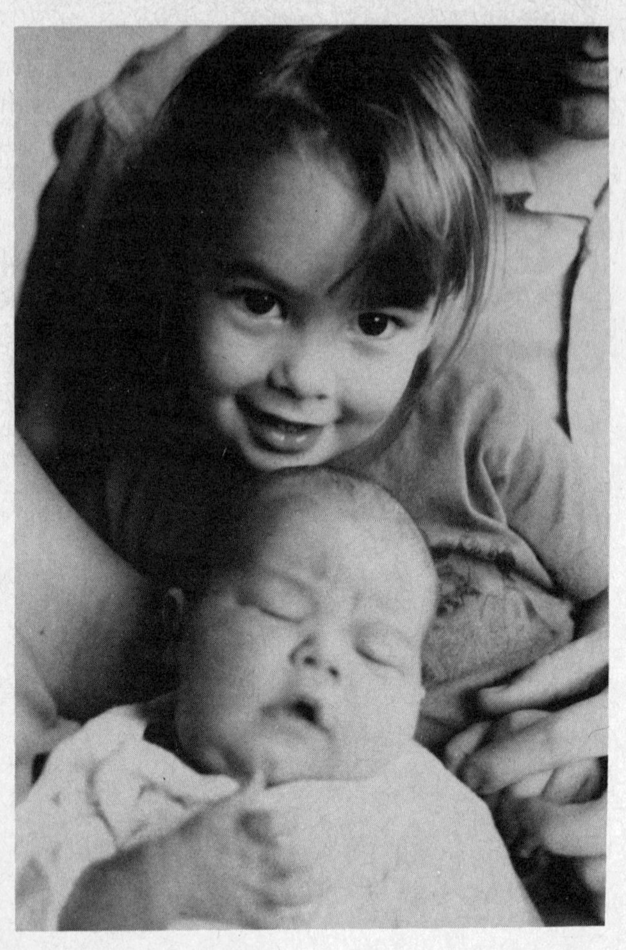

chapter three

How Unnecessary Cesareans Are Made

I once met an obstetrician who had recently moved to the United States from St. Thomas, which has a far lower cesarean rate. I asked him how he liked obstetrics in the States.

"It's wonderful!" he exclaimed.

"What do you mean?" I said, surprised at his enthusiasm. "Isn't childbirth pretty much the same the world over?"

"Not at all," he began. "Delivering babies can be quite boring in St. Thomas. It's always the same thing. We rarely see cesareans. But here I get to do cesareans all the time."

"Do you prefer cesarean surgery to spontaneous birth?"

"Yes!" he said. "It's much more exciting, more challenging!"

This attitude is not unusual. In fact, it is far more common than most parents realize. If one approaches birth as a medical event, a cesarean *is* more exciting than normal labor.

There is nothing like childbirth in America. We are the world's leader in cesarean surgery and all sorts of other obstetrical interventions. We are also one of the world's leaders in childbirth complications of almost every description, including the death of babies.

Nature designed mothers to give birth naturally. Genuine complications interrupting this marvelous process are rare. Why, then, are there so many surgical births?

The attitudes of a great many physicians discussed ahead in more detail is only one of the many reasons the U.S. cesarean rate is what it is. Actually, multiple factors lead to unnecessary cesareans. Trying to understand all these factors is like trying to play underwater chess with fogged goggles. At best, the answers are vague. However, acquainting yourself with the major factors that contribute to unnecessary surgery will help you make better birth plans and decrease your chance of surgical birth.

MAJOR CAUSES OF UNNECESSARY CESAREAN SURGERY

The following are the major factors contributing to otherwise avoidable cesarean birth. Some are discussed in this chapter and some in Chapter Four. With careful planning, you should be able to eliminate all of them.

- Negative beliefs about childbirth
- Injudicious use of medical intervention, including:
  - Regional anesthesia
  - Electronic fetal monitoring
  - Artificial rupture of the membranes
  - Augmentation of labor with Pitocin
  - Other medical intervention, including intravenous feeding

- A caregiver who has a high cesarean rate or with whom you are incompatible
- An environment incompatible with normal labor
- Poor nutrition during pregnancy
- Inappropriate use of health insurance

In certain unusual situations, you may not be able to avoid everything on this list. For example, if you have a medically complicated pregnancy or labor, you may require medical intervention. If this is the case, be especially careful about following all the rest of the steps in this book to lower your chance of cesarean birth.

THE MYTH THAT BIRTH IS A MEDICAL EVENT: NEGATIVE BELIEFS

Most cesarean mothers are victims of America's most widespread health myth: that birth is a medical event rather than a natural, normal part of life.

Childbirth has changed dramatically over the past few years. Women are treated more humanely than they were in 1970, when the cesarean rate was 5.5 percent. Yet the cesarean rate has quadrupled to its present 23 percent (and greater than 30 percent at some hospitals).

Though there is a widespread movement toward natural birth, home birth, alternative birth centers, and so forth, there is also an opposite pull toward increased technological intervention. The rigid policies of many hospitals still prevent mothers from having their own baby in the way they choose and with whom they choose present. In many institutions, a perfectly healthy mother is cast in a "sick" role with intravenous feeding, giving the impression that she was having a heart attack, not a baby. Comfortable birthing rooms have not yet replaced clinical-looking delivery rooms and stainless steel tables in some hospitals, despite the obvious influence environment has on labor. Behind the scenes is the underlying attitude woven like an insidious thread into the very fabric of American childbirth: birth is a medical crisis. This attitude, more than anything else, is at the root of America's appalling cesarean rate.

Labor is the only natural process that we have turned into a clinical procedure. Appropriate medical watchfulness is undeniably important for a safe outcome. Problems can and sometimes do occur that require expert intervention. However, this doesn't imply that normal birth is a medical event.

When you think of it, the practice of casting a woman at the very height of her creative power in a sick role is nothing less than fantastic. Yet what is even stranger is that parents *accept* this role. Though they claim to believe that childbirth is a natural process, many act as though it were an illness. And as long as mothers are separated from their families, isolated in sterile hospital rooms, and treated like invalids, we can expect the cesarean rate to continue to soar.

In the Netherlands, on the other hand, birth is viewed as the normal event it is. Midwives outnumber physicians, and training for midwifery does not require that one be a nurse, as it does in the United States. Home birth is widely accepted and encouraged, not frowned upon as it often is in the United States. The difference is striking. The Dutch rate of *episiotomy* (surgical incision to enlarge the birth outlet as the baby is born) is 6 percent compared to greater than 90 percent in the United States; the use of forceps and vacuum extraction in the Netherlands is 4 percent, and the cesarean rate is 5 percent.[1] Women in the Netherlands are not physically different from women in America, they only approach birth differently.

We can benefit from their example. Developing a positive view of birth (as discussed in the next chapter) and planning to be attended only by those who treat laboring women as healthy mothers rather than ill patients will lower your chance of surgical birth.

The attitudes of expectant parents as well as the practices of childbirth professionals must change dramatically before we will see a significant reduction in the cesarean rate. David Stewart, medical statistician and executive director of NAPSAC International (The National Association of Parents and Professionals for Safe Alternatives in Childbirth) believes that if good parental nutrition, natural childbirth and home birth were to become the norm, cesarean rates would fall to justifiable levels of less than 5 percent.

INJUDICIOUS USE OF MEDICAL INTERVENTION

A high percentage of cesarean sections—perhaps the overwhelming majority—are indirectly caused by physicians and hospitals. Inappropriate hospital procedures and unnecessary medical intervention interfere with normal labor. This in turn often leads to failure to progress and fetal distress, the most common indications for a primary cesarean.

Regional Anesthesia

In one hospital I visited, one in every four mothers opts for epidural anesthesia for normal labor. The cesarean rate at that hospital is over 30 percent.

According to Dr. John B. Caire of Lake Charles Memorial Hospital in Lake Charles, Louisiana, the use of regional anesthesia (epidural, spinal, caudal, saddleblock, and so forth) reduces labor's effectiveness, causes various degrees of *fetal anoxia* (inadequate oxygen supply), and hinders the bearing-down process.[2] Epidural anesthesia may be associated with an increased need for Pitocin and a higher rate of cesarean surgery. Additional disadvantages of regional anesthesia include an increased need for forceps delivery and, usually, more extensive episiotomy and lacerations.

Sometimes anesthesia is needed. However, for normal labor, alternatives are discussed in the section "Effective Labor Support" in Chapter Five. In addition, if you follow *all* of the steps in the next two chapters, your labor is likely to be shorter and less painful.

Electronic Fetal Monitoring (EFM)

The electronic fetal monitor (EFM) is a machine that records both fetal heart rate (FHR) and the intensity of uterine contractions on a continuous sheet of graph paper. There are two basic types of monitoring, external and internal.

External monitoring. Two straps, attached to a nearby machine, are placed around the mother's abdomen. On one, an ultrasound transducer picks up the FHR. On the other, a pressure-sensitive device detects the intensity of uterine contractions.

Internal monitoring. A wire is passed through the vagina and cervix and attached to the baby's scalp to pick up the FHR. A fluid-filled, pressure-sensitive catheter is also inserted into the uterus to determine the intensity of contractions. (Often the FHR is monitored internally and contractions are monitored externally.) Internal monitoring is more accurate but also more invasive.

Originally introduced to monitor high-risk labor, EFM has unfortunately become widespread and is routinely used in normal labor. In some hospitals, EFM is universal.

Since it plays a significant role in increasing the probability of a cesarean, EFM merits special attention here.

According to an NIH report about diagnostic methods, "Present evidence does not show benefit of electronic fetal monitoring to low-risk patients."[3]

The use of EFM (and this also applies to other medical intervention, including the use of routine IV) *disrupts normal labor.* It is, no doubt, for this reason that some medical studies have shown the cesarean rate for dystocia (impaired labor) to have doubled among electronically monitored mothers.[4]

EFM increases the probability of a cesarean in several ways:

1. Misinterpretation of monitor tracings: Monitors frequently malfunction, giving erroneous information. Often the person reading the tracings misunderstands their meaning. In fact, according to Dr. John B. Caire, external monitors are subject to an error of interpretation rate as high as 75 percent.[5]

2. The supine position often adopted during EFM leads to fetal oxygen deprivation.[6] This condition is exacerbated and may even be life threatening if the mother has epidural anesthesia.

3. Even if the mother doesn't lie on her back during labor, EFM does inhibit her mobility, which interferes with normal labor and may lead to fetal distress.[7] By the same token, the mother's partner is inhibited from providing the close, caressing labor support so helpful in cesarean prevention when she is hooked up to machines.

4. Internal EFM requires rupture of the membranes, which carries its own risks.

5. With a belt around her abdomen and a wire running out of her vagina, the mother's spontaneous reaction to

labor is severely inhibited. Drs. Howard L. Minkoff and Richard H. Schwartz have called attention to "the stress a monitored patient may experience because of the use of noisy, incomprehensible machines. Stress is associated with the release of catecholamines and their release may produce vasoconstriction and reduced utero-placental perfusion with heart rate decelerations."[8]

In an often-quoted study,[9] Dr. Albert Haverkamp and three other physicians divided 483 mothers of similar risk status into two groups. One group had EFM. In the other, a nurse listened to the FHR through a *fetoscope* (*auscultation*). Among the monitored mothers, *the cesarean rate was 2½ times higher, with no difference in the baby's well-being* (16.6 percent compared with 6.6 percent in the auscultated group). Apgar scores taken at one minute were similar in both groups. However, the five-minute Apgar scores were superior in the auscultated group. There was also a dramatic increase in postpartum infection among the EFM group. (Other studies have clearly revealed that monitoring increases maternal infection.)[10]

The results surprised Dr. Haverkamp. He admits, "We expected that the electronically monitored infants would be in better condition than those who were merely auscultated since signs of distress could be acted upon more speedily."[11] However, he discovered that, contrary to the beliefs of many conscientious obstetricians, EFM is "not associated with an improvement in perinatal outcome."

Dr. Haverkamp later conducted another study with 690 mothers. This time, he discovered that the cesarean rate was *three times higher in the monitored group* (17.6 percent compared to 5.6 percent).

Like Dr. Haverkamp, several other physicians have clearly demonstrated a correlation between use of EFM and increased cesareans.[12] In another study, a group of monitored mothers had a cesarean section rate of 16 percent compared to 7 percent among nonmonitored mothers.[13] According to Dr. John B. Caire, with routine EFM, cesarean section rates "have risen dramatically without measurable increase in fetal salvage."[14]

In addition to increased postpartum infection, other risks of EFM include the potential danger of ultrasound, fetal scalp abscesses, and accidents to the baby from internal monitor electrodes.

As common sense indicates, the sensitive laboring mother needs human support, not machines bleeping beside her. Dr. Haverkamp and his colleagues point out:

> Nursing attention to the gravida [pregnant woman] with respect to maternal comfort, emotional support, and "laying on of hands" could have a significant impact on the fetus . . . The authors have the impression that the reassuring psychological atmosphere created by personal nurse interaction and the absence of the recording machine in auscultated patients contributed to the excellent infant outcome in auscultated patients.[15]

Occasionally, the judicious use of EFM reveals genuine fetal distress and may have a valid place in the obstetrical care of unusual labors. However, innumerable monitored mothers have had cesareans as a result of ominous-appearing alterations of the FHR (supposedly indicative of asphyxia) recorded on the machine. One study shows that fetal heart alteration is a normal stress response to labor. According to Dr. Hugo Lagerkrantz of the Karolinski Institute, "A normal catecholamine release in response to maternal labor could account for the complex heartbeats in many fetuses."[16]

In cases of genuine asphyxia, there is an alteration of pH in the fetal blood. Accordingly, many physicians suggest combining EFM with fetal scalp blood sampling, as this makes monitoring far more accurate and reduces the risk of a cesarean for false readings. However, this procedure necessitates inserting a cone-shaped object into the vagina along with a thin tube to draw off a few drops of blood from the baby's scalp. Obviously, this invasive interference with labor should be reserved only for those with complications.

One can't help wondering how EFM approaches universal use in some maternity units. One reason is America's love of technology and gadgetry of every kind. Another is, perhaps, lowered labor costs; fewer nurses are needed in labor and delivery units. Added to this is a failure to appreciate the fact that *the mother must feel normal in order to labor normally.*

Meanwhile, the widespread use of EFM is not to be blamed solely on well-meaning physicians. Many expectant parents love the machine. "I was glad June was being monitored every minute," one father said. "It was great seeing the contractions recorded on a graph." One mother said, "It made me feel secure to have the machine ticking at my side." Scores of parents feel the same way. And the cesarean rate continues to climb.

However, if your goal is cesarean prevention, it is valuable to avoid electronic fetal monitoring.

Artificial Rupture of the Membranes (ROM), or Amniotomy

Often the membranes (bag of waters) are ruptured in early or mid-labor by the examiner's finger or by a long plastic hook shaped somewhat like a crochet needle. This is done to speed up labor and/or to attach an electrode for internal EFM. While the procedure is painless, it does carry several risks to mother and baby.

The amniotic fluid within the membranes provides a sterile environment and cushions the baby during uterine contractions so that pressure is evenly distributed. It may also serve other, as yet unknown functions. So at best it seems rather silly to rupture the membranes.

ROM very definitely increases the likelihood of surgical birth. In most hospitals, once the membranes are ruptured, the clock is set in motion. The mother is generally expected to give birth within twenty-four hours (to reduce the chance of infection) or she receives Pitocin to augment labor. In addition, after ROM, cord compression, and perhaps a fall in uterine blood flow, may contribute to fetal distress,[17, 18] which can and often does result in a cesarean.

Studies have shown that amniotomy can shorten labor by about an hour. However, other studies have suggested that the effect of artificial rupture of the membranes on the length of labor is inconsistent and unpredictable.[19] Dr. Roberto Caldeyro-Barcia, former president of the International Federation of Gynecologists and Obstetricians and director of the Latin American Center of Perinatology and Human Development for the World Health Organization, points out that "acceleration of labor is not necessarily beneficial for the fetus and newborn and that it may be associated with poor outcome for the offspring."[20]

During very late labor, some mothers find artificial ROM a relief. This, of course, should be left to the mother's choice. Meanwhile, there are other ways of shortening labor, such as assuming the vertical rather than the horizontal position[21] and having the effective support of your partner throughout (see Chapter Five).

Pitocin

Pitocin, an artificial form of the hormone oxytocin, which helps to regulate labor contractions, is often administered intravenously to induce an overdue labor or augment a flagging labor. This is recommended when labor does not progress on its own and there is no other way to get it going (see Chapter Five, the sections "If Your Labor Is Overdue" and "If Your Labor Stops or Slows Down"). However, Pitocin does carry several risks.

Pitocin-induced contractions are usually more tumultuous, less easy to manage. They seem to rise suddenly to a peak rather than building up gradually. This frequently creates a need for pain-relief medication. In addition, at most hospitals, mothers who have Pitocin must also have EFM.

The following is a typical scene often repeated in hospitals. The mother's labor stops or slows down—frequently as a result of emotional factors, perhaps her response to being hooked up to EFM. Pitocin is administered to augment contractions. This causes such painful contractions that the mother requires medication. The medication further slows her labor. The Pitocin dosage is increased. And so on the vicious cycle spirals until fetal distress is recorded on the monitor and the decision to do an "emergency" cesarean is made.

The Pitocin/cesarean scenario has many variations. However, as discussed in Chapter 5, there are many other ways to speed up labor that can be tried before resorting to Pitocin. Moreover, if you follow all the steps in the book, your labor will be less likely to be unnecessarily disturbed.

Other Injudicious Medical Intervention

Medical intervention of any kind, however minor, is inappropriate unless the mother has a medical complication requiring it. Therefore, the healthy mother should avoid all medical intervention. The following are the three most common procedures:

Intravenous feeding replaces normal consumption of fluid and food in some hospitals. Few will disagree that IVs play an important role in the treatment of sick persons, and that under some unusual circumstances they may even be justified during labor. However, hooking a normal, healthy mother-to-be to an IV is an utterly bizarre practice.

Those who favor the use of IVs during labor claim that the IV will make it easier to administer medication or an immediate blood transfusion if the mother requires it. If the mother is forbidden foods and liquids by mouth, the IV is needed to prevent dehydration or hypoglycemia. However, these reasons hardly justify routine intravenous feeding. The mother is far less likely to require medical intervention if she drinks and eats lightly to satisfy her body's needs.

Enemas are still commonly administered shortly after admission in a few hospitals, though for the most part this procedure is falling by the wayside. The enema clears the bowels prior to birth. However, prelabor diarrhea usually does this effectively. If not, the expression of a little stool, common during birth, is scarcely noticed by the birth attendants and simply wiped away.

Some mothers find the enema quite uncomfortable, especially if they are in advanced labor. Others prefer it. If so, a self-administered enema at home is usually the most comfortable.

Prepping refers to shaving the hair around the birth outlet, while miniprepping is clipping the hair, two other practices now falling by the wayside. Shaving the pubic hair makes the mother look and feel silly as well as causing discomfort during the postpartum period when the hair grows back. In the past, prepping was thought to reduce the chance of infection. However, this is not the case. In fact, it may even increase the possibility of infection.[22]

The best principle to observe in all obstetrical decisions is: *If it works, don't fix it. Otherwise it might really break down.*

Interference with normal labor profoundly influences the childbearing process in ways that cannot always be directly seen, as well as in the ways discussed above. As I emphasize in *Mind Over Labor,* "whatever affects the laboring mind affects the laboring body." The highly sensitive laboring mother can't avoid being influenced by the way her labor is managed. Her labor is not likely to function normally if she feels upset by interference, any more than lovemaking would function normally under similar conditions. Her hormonal balance is thrown off. Her uterine contractions may slow down or stop altogether. Her anxiety may be severe enough to cause fetal distress, necessitating more intervention.

All too often, the final scene is cesarean surgery.

THE HOSPITAL ENVIRONMENT

Another factor contributing to unnecessary surgery is the hospital environment. Fortunately, hospitals are changing for the better as a more humanistic maternity care evolves. However, many hospitals are still poor places for normal labor. Even if the mother feels safest and most secure giving birth in the hospital, the clinical setting of many institutions, the presence of strangers, and restrictive hospital policies are bound to make her feel inhibited.

The environment can disrupt labor in subtle ways that

are not apparent to most observers. For example, though not meaning to be insensitive, staff persons often make comments that hinder the labor process. A simple remark about the mother's "slow" labor or the fact that she doesn't seem to be making progress can actually impede normal labor by making her feel upset or inadequate. There is usually nothing abnormal about a "slow" labor. However, if the mother fears that her labor is abnormal and becomes upset about it, she may actually stop dilating.

Hospital birth is a matter of convention with sometimes little basis in logic. America's almost universal hospital birth is one of the strangest customs of modern times. Technology is so inextricably woven into the American consciousness that we have turned childbirth, the most natural of events, into a hospital procedure. Unfortunately, this practice has cost untold thousands of mothers unnecessary cesareans and unpleasant birth experiences.

American childbirth professionals, as well as parents, seem geared against childbirth at home (a fact that future generations will probably discount as too strange to be true). Horrifying as it sounds, there are many physicians who will refuse prenatal care to a mother planning a home birth. Anyone who refuses care for such a reason is, in my opinion, guilty of a far more serious form of malpractice than that for which most physicians are sued.

According to David and Lee Stewart, in *The Childbirth Activists' Handbook*, "Hospitals have never been proven to be the safest place for most women to give birth."[23] In fact, studies have shown quite the opposite. In a study conducted by Dr. Lewis Mehl comparing home birth with a similar number of hospital births among a matching population, in-hospital birth was associated with a greater rate of fetal distress, birth injury, infants with low Apgar scores, postpartum hemorrhage, neonatal infection, respiratory disease, and neurologically damaged infants. Cesarean rates were *nearly four times greater among the hospital births* (8.2 percent compared with 2.7 percent).

This doesn't mean that you have to give birth at home to avoid a cesarean. There are hospitals with environments conducive to normal labor, and of course there are childbearing centers. However, wherever you give birth, it is essential to avoid a high-cesarean environment, that is, a setting that by its very nature impairs normal labor. Human labor is hard enough as nature designed it without increasing the challenge with unnecessary obstacles.

Suggestions for choosing an environment conducive to normal childbirth are included in the next chapter.

Warning Signs of a High-Cesarean Environment

Avoid the following:

- Unsupportive or insensitive staff persons.
- Restrictive policies preventing the mother from eating or drinking to satisfy her body's desires, from moving around freely, from giving birth the way she chooses, from inviting the guests of her choice to share her experience, and so forth.
- Unnecessary noise from loudspeakers, etc. (Loudspeakers should not be on a maternity unit.)
- A clinical setting.
- An institution with a high cesarean rate.
- A setting that makes you feel uncomfortable.
- Lack of privacy

MALPRACTICE SUITS

Today, suits of every description are seen more and more often. We are becoming a sue-happy society in which it seems anyone can be sued for anything. When it comes to legal complications among physicians, obstetricians are particularly vulnerable. The likelihood that an obstetrician/gynecologist will be sued for malpractice is 2.4 times the average.[24]

Many obstetricians are justifiably afraid that if they don't do everything possible for a "perfect baby," including performing a cesarean section, they will be blamed and in for a malpractice suit. To avoid this, the obstetrician may perform a cesarean in the name of "defensive medicine." He can therefore prove that he did everything possible.

The exhaustive study by Dr. Helen Marieskind for the U.S. Department of Health, Education and Welfare claims that the threat of malpractice suits is the most significant factor in the rise of incidence of cesarean birth.[25] However, one cannot really determine precisely how much malpractice suits have affected the cesarean rate. In fact, as *Cesarean Childbirth* points out, in settings where physicians are not open to personal liability for malpractice, such as military and public health service hospitals, the cesarean rate has shown a comparable rise to that of physicians in private practice.[26]

Yet one cannot overlook the fact that malpractice suits *have* had an effect. Fear of malpractice is perhaps one of the greatest enemies of vaginal birth after cesarean. Thanks to the threat of suits, physicians are anxious to avoid deviating from currently accepted modes of practice—however much evidence may be in favor of new methods.

Suits frequently revolve around injuries to a baby occurring during or shortly after vaginal delivery, such as brain damage as a result of negligent use of forceps. Physicians have been sued for a poor outcome after a vaginal delivery if the parents believe the damage could have been avoided had a cesarean been performed. Yet the mode of delivery may have no relation to the infant's mortality or morbidity. Other malpractice suits focus on things that happened during surgery rather than failure to perform surgery. Families have won lawsuits because physicians delayed doing cesareans when the baby was thought to be at risk.[27]

Health-care consumers, therefore, as well as physicians, are responsible for the spiraling cesarean rate.

As Dr. Eugene C. Sandberg of Stanford, California, eloquently states:

> When there is uncertainty regarding the interpretation of the fetal heart rate pattern in labor, when there is uncertainty regarding whether the fetus presenting by the breech can successfully be delivered vaginally, when there is uncertainty regarding whether forceps manipulation should be undertaken, when there is uncertainty regarding whether bleeding or toxemia can be controlled long enough to permit vaginal delivery before fetal oxygenation is impaired (i.e., whenever one skirts the edge of an obstetric malresult), the safest and wisest course is to deliver by cesarean section without further deliberation.
>
> To persist in the attempt to obtain a living and normal neonate by vaginal delivery and, by using impeccable logic, extensive knowledge, broad experience, and perfect judgment, to win, gains one little. A good result was expected. To persevere and to fail to get a good neonatal result, even though those same godly qualities were at work, is a calamity. A malresult potentially subjects the obstetrician to the ridicule of his or her peers, the unhappiness of the patient and all of her family and friends, and frequently, the necessity to explain to a lay jury the nuances of obstetric judgment and the justification for fallibility. . . .
>
> To have avoided the challenge and to have opted,

> without further expenditure of time or thought, for cesarean section, and to have won, is to have performed to the standard expected.[28]

Not only does the obstetrician fear suit, he must also pay exorbitant insurance premiums. This is reflected in rising obstetrical fees. Therefore, malpractice suits ultimately hurt clients as well as physicians.

Possible solutions to this problem include greater physician/client communication; shared decision making; parents taking greater responsibility for their own birth experience; willingness to become well informed and choose one's options wisely; and realistic expectations and awareness of the limits of medical practice.

THE ATTITUDE OF MANY PHYSICIANS

As already stated, cesarean surgery has become increasingly safer for mother and baby (but by no means as safe as vaginal birth). Many physicians have adopted a somewhat casual attitude. They feel it doesn't really matter how the baby is born as long as mother and baby are healthy. They are often unaware of the far-reaching consequences of surgical birth trauma. Meanwhile, the criterion for surgical delivery has relaxed, making it easier for a physician to make the cesarean decision.

Cesarean section also carries a built-in financial incentive for the physician. Not only is his fee greater, but surgery takes less time—an hour compared with perhaps several hours for vaginal birth.

We would all like to believe that physicians are serving the interest of better health, not personal greed. Perhaps this is so with many doctors. However, according to a report published by the U.S. Department of Health and

Human Services, "The ratio of obstetricians to females of childbearing age has risen, suggesting a fall in average practice size, which, in turn, creates pressures to maintain practice income by opting for the more remunerative cesarean procedures."[29]

Several studies clearly show that the surgical birth rate varies with insurance coverage.[30] According to one study, the cesarean rate among patients with full coverage was 20.2 percent compared to 11.9 percent among those with no coverage.[31]

A California Department of Health Services study covering 1977–78 revealed that the cesarean rate in Medicaid recipients was 10.4 percent compared to a 15.4 percent rate for the entire state.[32]

Nationally, in 1983, the cesarean rate was 22.5 percent among Blue Cross patients, 21.5 percent among mothers with other private commercial insurance, 18.6 percent for Medicaid, 17.1 percent for self-payment, 16.7 percent for other government payment, and 11.4 percent for no charge. According to the American Journal of Public Health, this pattern is similar to that observed in several previous years.[33]

"If the desire is for a normal vaginal delivery," states Norbert Gleicher, M.D. in his article in the *Journal of the American Medical Association,* "One must conclude that it is preferable to have that delivery at a county teaching hospital, without insurance coverage."[34] Actually, the parents might even do better to have the baby at home or in a childbearing center.

INAPPROPRIATE USE OF HEALTH INSURANCE

When our own health insurance lapsed just before we discovered our first child was on the way, Jan and I were terribly disappointed. It was too late to reinstate. However, this turned out to be the best thing that could have happened to us. It would have been impossible to plan the wonderful birth we shared with the particular physicians and hospital our health insurance had provided for.

For many expectant parents, health insurance is the ticket to a free cesarean. Many health plans have arrangements with a particular hospital or group practice, a large number of whom have high cesarean rates. As mentioned above, studies have shown that the cesarean rate is much higher among insured mothers.

The problem lies not with health insurance itself but in the fact that many parents allow their insurance policy to determine where they will give birth and who will attend them. Health insurance, however, should *never* be the deciding factor in choosing a caregiver or birthing environment. Your choice of caregiver should always be based on compatibility. You should choose a birthing environment because you genuinely believe that it is the best place for you to begin your family.

As suggested above, many parents would be better off without health insurance when it comes to having a baby. According to the U.S. Department of Health and Human Services report, "Women with no insurance are least likely to receive a cesarean delivery."[35] The majority seem to take a decision more seriously when they are paying for it out of their own pocket.

This doesn't mean that you must cancel your health insurance to avoid a cesarean. However, you should not let your insurance influence your birth plans, even if it means losing the benefits of that insurance and incurring additional cost.

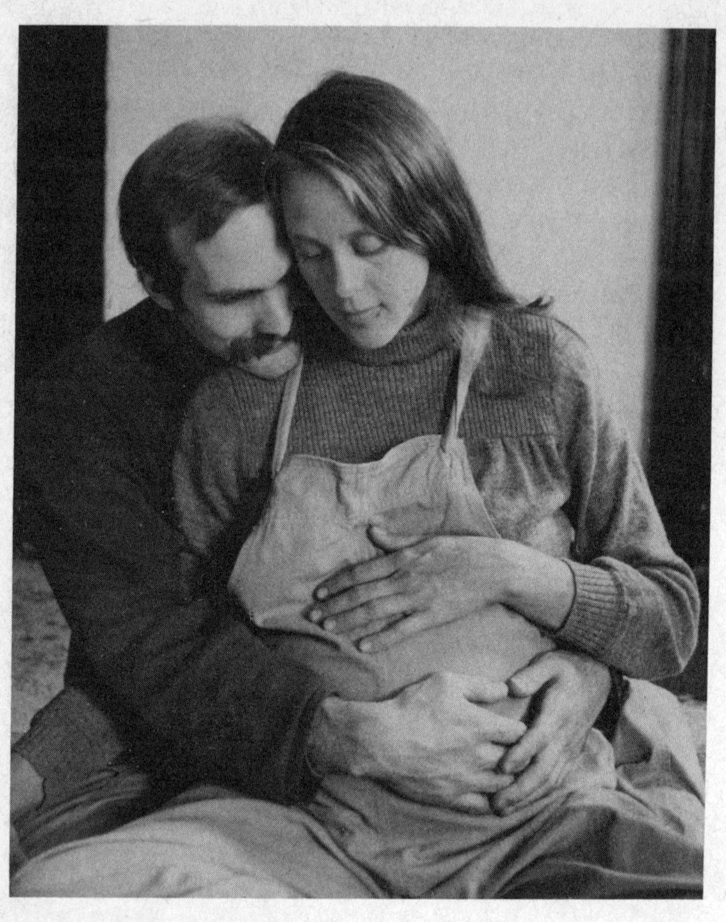

chapter four

Ten Steps to Cesarean Prevention: Pregnancy

No one can determine precisely how your labor will turn out—whether it will be long or short, or how it will feel, any more than one can accurately guess what your baby will look like by glancing at your belly. However, you can create the conditions for labor to unfold optimally by following the ten steps in this chapter.

Observing the practical guidelines in this and the following chapter will increase your chance of birthing normally dramatically. Very probably, these simple steps will also decrease the length of your labor by eliminating obstacles to efficient childbearing such as a poor birthing environment.

The steps ahead *will* help you prevent an unnecessary cesarean. But in order to be truly effective, you must not omit a single one of them.

CESAREAN PREVENTION: A JOINT EFFORT

Prepare for birth with your partner. Though it is the mother who bears the child, preventing a cesarean is as much the father's responsibility as it is hers. Couples who share pregnancy and plan childbearing together are far more likely to share a fulfilling birth.

Besides, the father should be thoroughly acquainted with the essentials of cesarean prevention so that together he and his partner can make appropriate birth plans and so that he can give more effective support during labor. He should take part in all major decisions, from choosing a caregiver to making contingency plans should a cesarean be necessary.

TAKING RESPONSIBILITY

The key to effective cesarean prevention is taking responsibility for your birth experience. No one can do this for you. You can't depend on a caregiver or a childbirth educator to insure that you will avoid a cesarean. Only you can create the optimal birth experience.

You create your birth much more so than most parents realize. Your attitudes about childbirth and the birth plans you make shape your birth experience, including whether or not you have a cesarean. They even influence the postpartum experience—days, weeks, sometimes months after birth. This is especially so in a country with so many birthing options.

You may think that expectant parents should be able to trust their local hospital and caregiver, believing that they must know their business. However, there are numerous options available, and many styles of obstetrical practice. The way labor is approached and women are treated differ from one birthing institution to another. Some caregivers and birthing places support natural birth, others have very high cesarean rates.

Over the past few decades, American obstetrics has gone haywire. The very fact that 750,000 American mothers give birth via major abdominal surgery every year, and that having a baby at home is practically illegal in some states, is evidence of a species of madness perhaps unparalleled in any other field. We are just beginning to emerge from an obstetrical dark age. New childbearing customs are evolving, and in the future, they will perhaps replace the bizarre childbearing customs of our day. For example, more and more childbirth professionals and parents have come to appreciate the safety and practicality of home birth for healthy mothers. Midwifery is seeing a renaissance. Some hospitals offer environments suitable for beginning a family—a room or suite where the family can share the childbearing miracle and remain together afterward until discharge. However, at this point in obstetrical history, childbirth in America is still characterized by some strange rites and practices.

For this reason, it is essential that you plan your birth cautiously.

Some parents believe that they have no choices, that their insurance pays for a particular institution, and so forth. But there are almost always options.

Bear in mind that giving birth is one of the biggest events of your life. Do everything in your power to make it special. You, your partner, and your baby will never regret that you did.

THE TEN ESSENTIAL STEPS

The ten essential cesarean prevention steps to follow during pregnancy are:

1. Get good nutrition.
2. Exercise regularly.
3. Understand labor.
4. Examine your beliefs.
5. Develop positive attitudes and beliefs about birth.
6. Plan your birth.
7. Choose a compatible caregiver.
8. Choose a birthing place conducive to normal labor.
9. Prepare for effective labor support.
10. Make contingency plans.

Each of these will be discussed in turn. The next chapter covers preventive steps to observe during labor. It should also be read now. Many suggestions in Chapter Five require prenatal preparation.

It is best to begin preparing for birth early in pregnancy. However, it is never too late—even if you are reading this book on your due date. My wife Jan and I thought we had planned our first birth well, only to discover when Jan went into hard labor that our physician was away for the weekend. We hadn't met the physician's back-up to see whether or not we agreed with his policies and were compatible, a foolish oversight. So when contractions were coming every three minutes, we made a frantic last-minute decision to change both physicians and hospitals. At 3:30 A.M. we called another physician we knew and asked him to attend our birth. I doubt we could have shared the wonderful birth experience we did if we hadn't made the last-minute change.

GET GOOD NUTRITION

"There are no safe alternatives in childbirth without good nutrition in pregnancy," state David and Lee Stewart in *The*

Childbirth Activists' Handbook.[1] Good nutrition is the basis of prenatal health and a safe birth. A host of complications can be avoided by eating a well-balanced diet throughout the pregnant months.

Getting good nutrition also implies avoiding junk foods (highly processed or empty-calorie foods). The expectant mother who smokes should eliminate smoking, even if this is difficult for her. Smoking impairs fetal growth and is associated with several complications of childbirth.

You should also moderate the use of alcohol. Heavy drinking can seriously damage the baby, leading to a combination of physical and mental disorders known as *fetal alcohol syndrome.* No one knows the precise limits of safe alcohol consumption, and many childbirth professionals feel it is best to eliminate it completely. However, the majority believe a small amount is not harmful.

EXERCISE REGULARLY

Prenatal exercise does not directly influence uterine contractions. However, many mothers do seem to have shorter labors if they have exercised regularly throughout pregnancy. Besides, common sense suggests that a woman in good physical condition is more likely to birth normally than a woman in poor shape.

Throughout pregnancy, you can continue any safe physical activity to which your body is already accustomed. However, don't begin any *new* strenuous activity.

Avoid jarring movements, since your body's connective tissues are loosened as a result of hormones. Also avoid exercise that may cause you to lose balance, as your center of gravity is altered during the prenatal months.

The best all-around exercise is walking. Throughout our three pregnancies, my wife and I hiked in the mountains, our favorite outdoor activity. This kept us both in shape and justified the oftentimes huge meals we ate.

Other aerobic exercises beneficial during pregnancy are swimming and bicycling. Strenuous aerobics like long-distance running and water skiing are discouraged.

UNDERSTAND LABOR

All childbirth classes and most books about birth cover the physical aspects of labor. But in addition to knowing the basics of how labor works physically, you should be acquainted with the *inner event of labor,* an idea introduced in *Mind Over Labor.* This refers to two fundamental ideas: the laboring woman's altered state of mind and the sexuality of childbirth. Understanding the inner event of labor is the key to making appropriate birth plans. It will go further toward reducing your chance of an unnecessary cesarean than all the other steps in this book combined. In fact, if parents planned their birth with the inner event of labor in mind and were taught to develop a positive view of birth, I believe we would see a dramatic reduction in the cesarean rate.

The body and the mind cannot be separated during childbearing. The way the mother feels and thinks, as well as her birthing environment, all profoundly influence uterine function. Childbearing—more than any other physical process except, perhaps, lovemaking—is influenced by emotion. If a woman is tense, anxious, or feels she is not in a suitable place to give birth, her labor can and often does slow down or stop altogether. Emotional factors are often the indirect, but nonetheless real, cause of surgical birth.

The Laboring Woman's Altered State of Mind

During early labor, the mother may be excited, talkative, anxious, or a bit of each, or she may act and feel pretty much her ordinary self. But as labor progresses, she experiences a profound psychological change.

As labor rolls along, the right hemisphere of the brain dominates the scene. This hemisphere, sometimes referred to as the *heart brain,* is associated with intuition, lovemaking, emotion, and labor. Meanwhile, the left hemisphere, associated with logic and rational thinking, seems to become less active.

The laboring mother seems to go into a world of her own. Her focus of concentration narrows dramatically. She becomes more introspective, focused only on her contractions and her partner. She gradually becomes wholly caught up in the force that will bring her baby into the world.

During late labor, she becomes an instinctive, primitive being. She is almost invariably less rational and more emotional. She is also highly sensitive and vulnerable. It is at this time that she needs her partner's nurturing support and to be in a peaceful, loving environment. Because the mind so dramatically affects uterine contractions, a positive emotional climate is essential for normal uterine function. A disturbance in the environment can impair labor and even precipitate the need for surgical birth.

Whatever affects the laboring mind affects the laboring body. Labor is impaired by emotional factors just as surely as a man often loses an erection in response to adverse emotional stimuli. Anything that disturbs the laboring mother's altered state of mind can create tension, upset her hormonal balance, and disrupt her labor.

Toward the climax of the childbearing drama, when the

cervix is dilating those final centimeters, the laboring woman very often becomes uninhibited, uttering sounds much like those of a woman nearing sexual climax. She sometimes removes all of her clothing, unconcerned about who sees her naked body. This is particularly common during childbearing-center and home births.

In my opinion, she also becomes radiantly beautiful toward labor's end. It is as if she has crossed the bridge from her everyday self to connect with her vast creative power capable of bringing forth a new life into the world.

The Sexuality of Labor

At first, you may think it odd that anyone would draw an analogy between lovemaking and labor contractions, which are often hard work and painful. However, the similarities between the two processes are more obvious when one notes the following:*

1. Labor takes place within the sexual organs.
2. The hormone oxytocin, is released during both lovemaking and labor. Oxytocin also helps to regulate breastfeeding. It is released when the mother is relaxed and in a safe, peaceful environment.
3. The uterus contracts rhythmically, though the intensity of contractions is far greater during labor.
4. Sensory acuity and awareness of the outer environment diminish toward the end of labor and toward sexual climax.
5. Intense emotions are experienced.

* This list is an expanded version of Niles Newton's comparison between lovemaking and labor in *Maternal Emotions.*[2]

6. Women usually become highly sensitive and vulnerable.

7. An expression of physical exertion appears on a woman's face near orgasm and during childbirth.

8. The mother often moans, sighs, and groans.

9. The mother's inhibitions decrease.

10. Both can be impaired by inhibitions, by negative attitudes, and by unfavorable conditions in the environment.

11. Both labor and lovemaking work optimally when the woman surrenders her mind and body to the process, when she allows instinct to take over.

The way a woman feels about sexuality, many childbirth professionals agree, is related to the way she labors. Mothers who are able to express themselves uninhibitedly in lovemaking are more likely to surrender to the unfamiliar sensations of labor. The mother who is sexually repressed, on the other hand, is likely to take her repression into the birthing room. In fact, feeling comfortable with one's sexuality is so essential that one maternity text stresses the need for the nurse to come to terms with her own sexuality so she can better help laboring women.[3]

Of course, this doesn't mean that every woman with a long or complicated labor is sexually repressed or that every woman with an unresolved sexual conflict is going to have a cesarean. It simply suggests that appreciating one's sexuality is a long step toward a rewarding birth. After all, labor and birth take place within the sexual organs. It stands to reason that one who appreciates this part of the anatomy as well as the experience of sexuality can better appreciate and cope with the childbearing miracle.

Normal birth is the flowering of the mother's sexuality—the height of her creative magic. Keeping this in mind rather than viewing birth as a medical crisis may reduce anxiety and help you yield to the labor process.

Viewing birth as a sexual event can also help the father give more effective labor support. With the sexual nature of birth in mind, for example, he understands why caressing and holding his partner can often be more effective than coaching her with breathing patterns. The father can help his partner surrender to labor by speaking to her in a soft, encouraging, loving voice, by touching her, and above all by just being there and sharing his love.

To prevent unnecessary surgery, it is essential to create conditions that support the inner event of labor. Otherwise, labor may not function optimally, and the likelihood of surgical birth is greater. What are those optimal conditions in addition to safety for mother and baby? *The same conditions that support satisfying lovemaking support normal labor.* Keep this in mind when you make your birth plans, and you will avoid many mistakes.

Without realizing it, expectant parents often throw obstacles in the way of normal birth by making plans that impair the inner event of labor, such as choosing an overly clinical birthing environment or an incompatible caregiver.

Imagine trying to enjoy satisfying lovemaking under conditions similar to those where women are expected to labor normally. The very thought would strike most people as absurd. Picture two lovers with IVs in their arms trying to have a go at it in a brightly lit, tiled room with clocks ticking, machines clicking, masked attendants milling about wearing sterile gloves, sterile drapes over the lovers' legs so only the genitals remain revealed, and perhaps someone commenting, "My, you folks are awfully slow, aren't you?"

This comparison may strike you as ridiculous. However, it is no more ridiculous than the way most American mothers give birth.

The "medicalization" of childbirth does more than interfere with labor on a physical plane. It disrupts the inner event of labor. It robs the mother of her sense of wholeness, her inner strength. It cuts her off from her connection with the universe, the very source of life.

The laboring mother is at once powerful, frail, and vulnerable as a newly blossoming flower. It is impossible to interfere with the course of a process so delicate and life-altering as human labor without adverse effects.

Helping childbearing women can only succeed as a health profession, I believe, when childbirth professionals recognize the inner event of labor. One of the most incredible anomalies about modern obstetrics is the almost complete ignorance of the way the mind influences labor. Some midwives and physicians have an intuitive understanding of the inner event of labor. Some caregivers have an "opening presence," that is, their personality and the way they behave around laboring women encourages them to relax, have confidence, and surrender to labor. However, astounding as it may seem, many physicians, midwives, maternity nurses, and childbirth educators know very little about the profound influence emotions have on uterine contractions, in spite of the fact that this is one of the most obvious characteristics of childbearing.

It is therefore up to you to create the conditions for the inner event of labor to unfold. By so doing, you will dramatically decrease your chance of surgical birth.

In addition, keep the following characteristics of labor in mind:

• Every labor is unique. Your labor may be wholly unlike the labors you've heard and read about.

• Labor varies in length from mother to mother. The average lengths of first and second stage cited in many books are just that—averages. A longer or shorter labor is by no means abnormal.

• For most mothers, labor is painful at times. However, labor is not all pain and struggle—it includes a wide range of feelings, from discomfort to ecstasy. For many women, labor is a richly rewarding experience. In addition, labor's pain can be mitigated with effective labor support, a positive attitude about birth, and a comfortable birthing environment.

EXAMINE YOUR BELIEFS

Next to good nutrition and understanding labor, this section and the following one, "Develop Positive Beliefs and Attitudes About Birth," are probably the most important but most often overlooked steps toward a normal birth. The way a woman feels about becoming a mother and about childbirth in general will affect her labor. As Joanna Sullivan Marut, R.N., points out in an article in the *American Journal of Maternal-Child Nursing,* "A woman's entire emotional past plays a vital role in determining the course of her labor."[4]

Obviously, beliefs alone are not responsible for the rising number of cesareans. The cesarean rate has quadrupled over the past two decades despite a generally improved attitude about birth. However, our beliefs and attitudes do influence our birth experience perhaps more than any other factor. According to psychotherapist Claudia Panuthos, author of *Transformation Through Birth,* cesarean mothers tend to believe that birth is unsafe or dangerous. "Difficult and complicated deliveries," she points out, "tend to support internal beliefs about birth and about the physical body."[5]

The notion that birth is dangerous, for example, triggers an instinctive urge to hold back in order to protect either infant or mother from harm. Meanwhile, one's negative views toward birth can be exacerbated by a lack of peace and harmony in the birthing environment.

Your feelings about your body are also reflected in your birth experience. Many childbirth professionals have observed that the mother who is comfortable with her body is more likely to birth normally.

A mother can unconsciously hold her labor back if she mistrusts her body or if she harbors a sufficiently strong negative view about birth. This, in turn, may trigger fetal and maternal complications leading to a cesarean. As Nancy Wainer Cohen and Lois Estner point out in *Silent Knife,* "The fact that our beliefs, our thoughts about ourselves, affect our births helps to explain, for example, why many women with an 'inadequate' or questionable pelvis give birth to 8-, 9-, or 10-pound infants, while other women with totally adequate pelves have difficulty or are unable to deliver their 6½- to 7-pound babies."[6]

Cesarean mothers frequently believe—sometimes unconsciously—that they *deserved* to have a cesarean. One mother, for example, felt she didn't deserve a normal birth in retribution for a prior abortion.

A cesarean is often the final symptom of the destructive belief, held by both parents and childbirth professionals, that medically managed labor is better than natural childbirth. Unnecessary cesareans are frequently the end result of the myth that technology is the best way to handle labor. In the final analysis, it boils down to a lack of trust in nature, in the female body, and in the childbearing process.

Explore your beliefs and attitudes. These stem from a variety of sources—your childhood, what you have learned from your mother and other relatives, stories you have heard, religious teaching, books, films, TV and so forth. If you find that your beliefs about birth and the body are predominantly negative (as are many American women's), examine them, do the best you can to let the negative ones go, and replace them with positive beliefs. Just becoming aware of negative beliefs and attitudes can lessen their power over your reactions.

Obviously, you can't simply erase your past. Don't expect to change all your attitudes about birth and the body over night. However, everything you do toward developing a positive view will help.

Meanwhile, you can create the other conditions for birth to progress optimally by following the remaining steps in this book.

DEVELOP POSITIVE ATTITUDES AND BELIEFS ABOUT BIRTH

In *Mind Over Labor,* I refer to a positive attitude about birth as "the cornerstone of a safe, happy, birth experience."[7] Developing a positive view is an essential step for anyone who wants to avoid unnecessary surgery.

This doesn't mean painting a rosy picture for yourself that denies the reality of pain in labor. However, it does mean eliminating the notion that birth is a medical crisis.

It is essential to accept childbearing as a natural, normal event.

One of the best ways to do this is to give yourself a realistic picture of labor. Understanding the inner event of labor is the first step. It is also helpful to widen your perspective of the childbearing miracle. Bear in mind that labor is the biggest social event in the lives of most couples—the beginning of a family. Think of your birth as you would your wedding, and plan accordingly. Most cesarean parents plan their births far more poorly than they would their wedding.

Also remember that you are the center of the childbearing drama. It is your birth, your baby, not your caregiver's or the hospital's. As you begin to assume responsibility and make plans compatible with normal birth, you feel less helpless, more in charge. Most likely you'll also find yourself developing a positive view of childbearing almost automatically.

Meanwhile, take time to admire the body and the amazing changes pregnancy brings. Have a warm, relaxing bath. Ask your partner to massage you. Above all, remind yourself that your changing body is beautiful. This is no exercise in self-deception. The changing prenatal shape really is beautiful. In ancient times, the prenatal form inspired nameless artisans to fashion goddess figures in the shape of expectant mothers—symbols of women's awesome ability to bring forth a new life.

Finally, take time to thank your body for the miracle it is now working and will continue to work. Your body is now accomplishing something as awesome as the creation of the earth. Your baby has developed from a single cell. The uterus has expanded to become her warm and secure home, her own private universe. It seems almost magical.

What is labor by comparison? Labor merely opens the door.

PLAN YOUR BIRTH

As long as parents plan their birth without first exploring their options, as do the majority of American couples, they remain at high risk of surgical birth. When a cesarean is performed, nine times out of ten the problem is to be found not in the mother's body or in the labor process but in her birth plans. The plans she has made, or failed to make—including choosing her caregiver and birthing place—can be her own worst enemy.

Many justifiably blame doctors, hospitals, and conventional obstetrics for the high cesarean rate. But when you come right down to it, the parents mold their own birth. Few are held prisoner by the medical establishment or are forced to give birth in a certain way or in a certain place. Almost everywhere, there are choices, alternatives.

Plan your birth as thoroughly as you are able and make contingency plans in the event of unforeseen complications.

ESSENTIALS TO INCLUDE IN YOUR BIRTH PLANS

Choice of caregiver

Choice of birthing place

Options of coping with labor

How you will cope with labor

How the father will participate during labor

Additional persons (if any) to be invited to share the birth: an additional labor-support person, family, friends, your children

How you will feed your baby (breast or bottle)

Your baby's medical care shortly after birth

Length of your hospital stay
Help at home after birth
What to do if there is an emergency

Explore your options. Get as many ideas as you can. Then decide what is most important to you. If something is essential to you, and you will not compromise about it, then this, of course, takes priority over less important elements in your plans.

You should not have to compromise about your own birth experience. However, you may have to go out of your way to achieve your goals. Many couples have temporarily relocated for the sake of a caregiver and birth place fully supportive of their plans.

Once you have a clear outline of your plans in mind or on paper, choose or evaluate your caregiver and birthing environment in light of these plans. Be sure your caregiver is aware of and fully supportive of your birth plans.

Always be open to making changes. For example, when you learn about the inner event of labor and discover the way environment influences the childbearing process and can contribute to unnecessary cesareans, you may find that your choice of birthing place is incompatible with normal labor. It is therefore appropriate to change plans.

Plan ahead about how the father will participate. If the father is not able to be actively involved giving labor support, be sure to have someone else perform this essential role.

Some men want to "catch" their own baby in addition to giving labor support. If the father wants to deliver his own child, the caregiver will usually manage the birth of the head—the part that most needs expert supervision.

Other fathers will prefer to cut the umbilical cord,

something I strongly recommend every father do. Cord-cutting (painless to baby and mother) can be a deeply meaningful ceremonial gesture, like placing the ring on the bride's finger.

Choose a Compatible Caregiver

Imagine hiring a painter to redo your living room. You have chosen the color—robin's-egg blue. It is a color you have liked since childhood. However, the painter refuses to accommodate. He tells you brusquely that he uses only bright red or shocking pink in living rooms. Would you pay this man to paint your room? No sane person would. Yet this is precisely the way a large percentage of women relate to their caregiver. They continue to visit a caregiver with whose policies they do not agree. All too frequently, a woman who claims to want a natural birth makes repeated appointments with a caregiver who has a high cesarean rate. This is not only absurd, it jeopardizes her birth experience.

Your likelihood of a cesarean is more than cut in half by choosing a compatible caregiver. On the other hand, your chance of surgical birth rises dramatically if you continue to visit a caregiver with whom you are incompatible or who has a high cesarean rate.

Most expectant mothers choose their caregivers more or less unconsciously. They select a physician or midwife because they assume the person is competent. However, there is far more than competence to be considered when it comes to inviting someone to share your most intimate family event.

Since you are not ill, but rather a woman on the threshold of motherhood, the patient/physician relationship is not an appropriate model in childbearing. Always think of yourself as a client, not a patient. When you hire a caregiver, you are paying a professional to perform a service. You have every reason to expect the service performed as you wish.

A number of health professionals give prenatal care and attend birth: obstetricians; family practitioners (physicians practicing general medicine and giving health care to the whole family); certified nurse midwives, or CNMs (persons trained in both nursing and midwifery and certified by the American College of Nurse Midwives); midwives trained through a midwifery school or through apprenticeship (often called "lay midwives" or simply "midwives"); and in some areas chiropractors and naturopaths.

As a general rule, your likelihood of surgical birth will drop significantly if you choose a midwife rather than an obstetrician. Because they are better trained in surgical procedure, obstetricians are more likely to opt for cesareans. In fact, the increasing number of mothers who choose obstetricians rather than family practitioners or midwives is one of the factors contributing to the rise in cesareans.[8] However, this by no means implies that you should rule out a sensitive caregiver simply because he or she is an obstetrician.

Midwives are often more noninterventive birth attendants than obstetricians. However, some obstetricians work with the souls of midwives, and many midwives work with clinical hands. I've met several wonderful physicians who are every bit as sensitive and noninterventive as the best midwives. I've also met insensitive midwives. Bear in mind that CNMs are part of the medical profession just as surely as are obstetricians, and choosing a midwife doesn't guarantee a noninterventive approach to labor.

Some religiously believe that women make better birth

attendants than men. A few books emphasize this notion in no uncertain terms. However, this is a myth. Both men and women can make equally good physicians, midwives, maternity nurses, and labor-support persons. Both can be equally nurturing. "Whether you're a childbirth educator, labor-support person, or midwife," states CNM Richard Jennings of Methodist Hospital in Philadelphia, "the important thing is not being male or female but having respect and wonderment for the birth process."

Of course, the gender of your caregiver is important if this matters to you.

Let your intuition be your guide when choosing a caregiver. Your "gut reaction" (in addition to the guidelines ahead) is often the best yardstick.

Both parents should take part in choosing the caregiver, and both should be comfortable with the person they are inviting to share the intimate birth experience. The father should also attend prenatal appointments with his partner. He doesn't have to be present at every single one, but he certainly should attend a few. The time he takes off from work, if the caregiver doesn't have evening hours, will prove well worth it. The advantages of father-attended prenatals are numerous: the parents choose or evaluate their caregiver together; the father is more involved in the pregnancy; his presence during prenatal appointments often makes the mother less nervous; sharing appointments puts the relationship with the caregiver in perspective, reminding the couple that the mother is a client experiencing a perfectly natural process—not an ill patient; the father is able to ask questions and air his own concerns; he will be less nervous giving support during labor if he is already acquainted with the caregiver.

Bear the following points in mind when choosing a

caregiver. If you already have a physician or midwife, use these points to evaluate your current caregiver:

- His or her cesarean rate. Avoid a caregiver with a high cesarean rate. What is high? In my opinion, anything over 6 percent is too high unless the practitioner specializes in high-risk pregnancy. However, most expectant parents are fortunate to find a caregiver with a 10 percent rate. If you have trouble finding a supportive physician with a low cesarean rate, get in touch with the Cesarean Prevention Movement, which has chapters nationwide and which has contact persons who are aware of local alternatives.
- Total support of your birth plans. Once you have finalized your plans, inform your caregiver of the details. If your physician or midwife refuses to go along with an important item, rule out that caregiver. And be sure your caregiver doesn't just "go along" with you to be agreeable. He should be fully supportive.
- A flexible approach to birth, not a "one-size-fits-all" obstetrical policy.
- Genuine support of natural childbirth. Many caregivers claim to support natural birth to accommodate their clients and then use unnecessary medical intervention through labor. Some will agree to do an episiotomy only if necessary, yet almost invariably find it "necessary."

Above all, remember: *It is never too late to change caregivers, and it is always better to change than continue visiting someone with whom you are incompatible.* If you can't find a caregiver with whom you are totally comfortable, be sure the person you choose supports the *major* elements in your birth plans. It is also wise to provide him with a written copy of your plans.

In addition, you and your partner can request to be alone together through most of labor.

If you plan a home birth and can't find a good caregiver to attend you, consult NAPSAC's *Directory of Alternative Birth Services* for the name of a qualified childbirth professional near your home. (See the suggested reading list at the end of this book.)

CHOOSE A BIRTHING PLACE CONDUCIVE TO NORMAL LABOR

Safety is, of course, the first concern when selecting a birthing place. Obviously, you want to be sure you and your baby will receive the best possible care.

Generally speaking, the safest birthing place is the environment in which you feel most comfortable—unless there are unusual medical complications requiring a hospital birth. For many, this is a hospital; for others, it is a childbearing center or home.

"A woman should give birth when, where and how she feels safe," says Esther Zorn, founder of the Cesarean Prevention Movement. "As a result of the instinctual nature of birth, if she doesn't feel way down deep that she is safe, her chances of having a positive birth experience are reduced."

Some hospitals with a peaceful atmosphere and a noninterventive staff that supports natural birth offer environments conducive to normal labor. However, many—if not most—have environments inimical to the childbearing process. The atmosphere is frequently riddled with interruptions, noise, clinical trappings, and the presence of unwanted strangers, all of which can impair labor's progress. As soon as you walk through the door of such an institution, your chance of surgical birth quadruples.

One study showed that hospitals with medical-school affiliations often perform more cesarean deliveries than other hospitals, and those with neonatal intensive care units frequently have the highest rates of all.[9]

"How much does it mean to you to avoid a cesarean?" Nancy Cohen, author of *Silent Knife* asks her clients. If it means a lot to them, her advice is simple. "Stay away from a birthing environment where surgery is done!"

For those who are uncomfortable with home birth yet don't want to labor in a hospital, the childbearing center is often the solution. Well-staffed childbearing centers offer excellent medical care with almost the comfort of home. For a list of birth centers nearest your home, write or call the National Association of Childbearing Centers. (See Resources.)

When selecting (or evaluating) your birthing place, keep the following in mind:

- Avoid a birthing place with the characteristics of a high-cesarean environment. In a high-cesarean environment, you are more likely to birth surgically regardless of your health and your baby's.
- Visit the birthing place. Preferably, visit several. Get a sense of the environment by talking with the staff, and follow your intuition. Never judge a hospital birthing room on the basis of a brochure!
- If you are planning a hospital birth, find out what its cesarean rate is before making a final choice. You put yourself at high risk of surgery if you labor in a hospital with a high cesarean rate.
- The cesarean rate is public information to which

you have a right. Ask your physician or the hospital staff. If you are planning a vaginal birth after a previous cesarean, find out about the repeat cesarean rate, if possible.

• Choose as nonclinical a setting as possible. The clinical atmosphere can cause labor to slow down, predisposing you to both medical intervention and complications leading to a cesarean.

• If you plan a hospital birth, be sure the hospital has a birthing room and encourages its use. In some hospitals where a birthing room is unavailable, you may be able to both labor and give birth in a labor room. However, in a few hospitals mothers are still routinely moved to a sterile delivery room when birth is imminent. This is not only a ludicrous childbearing custom, but it is physically and emotionally traumatic to the family unit. Besides, the delivery room is about as appropriate a place to begin a family as a gas station is to hold a wedding.

• Birthing rooms, by the way, are often used as an advertising gimmick. Before you choose a hospital for its birthing room, be sure that it is backed by a noninterventive staff and that you are not treated like an invalid within its walls.

• Be sure that the staff at your birthing place is used to mothers laboring without EFM and *encourages* this. Today's obstetrical professionals are actually losing the ability to watch normal birth carefully. As Dr. Albert Haverkamp points out: "Many nurses and doctors so rely on the electronic monitors that they feel lost without them."[10]

• Some hospital staff persons actually make a mother feel guilty if she doesn't use EFM—as if she were not concerned about her baby's welfare. This is particularly idiotic since those who refuse EFMs have often done extensive research about their options and want the best birth possible. If you choose a hospital where the majority are monitored, you set yourself up for an uncomfortable encounter as well as put yourself at high risk for a cesarean.

• Don't be misled by the expression "Family-Centered Maternity Care" (FCMC). While it is an important concept, the term is often used in advertisements to draw in clients. Yet some of the worst hospitals I have ever visited called themselves FCMC facilities.

• Choose a hospital that welcomes fathers during cesarean birth on the off chance that a cesarean is necessary. Most do. But some do not. No parent should support an institution that prohibits a father from attending the birth of his own child.

By asking questions of hospital administrators, physicians, and nurses, you are not only finding out vital information to plan your own birth. You are also helping to inspire much-needed changes in maternity care. It is especially important for consumers to require hospitals to disclose information about their cesarean rates. As more consumers do this, we will begin to see changes. In 1985, Massachusetts passed a law sponsored by C/SEC (a Boston-based group for cesarean prevention and emotional support for cesarean parents). It requires hospitals to give maternity patients information about the annual rate of primary cesareans, repeat cesareans, and percentage of women who have had vaginal births after a previous cesarean, in addition to other pertinent information. It is hoped that all states will eventually have similar laws.

MAKING CONTINGENCY PLANS

Though you should plan for and expect a natural vaginal birth, it is always wise to make emergency plans just in case a cesarean is necessary.

Read the final chapter and learn about your options regarding cesarean childbirth. Be aware of the choices of anesthesia, of the father's all-important role during and after surgical delivery, and of your options for postpartum care. If a cesarean is necessary, these issues can make all the difference in the world.

If you plan a home birth, choose a back-up hospital on the off chance of a last-minute transfer.

TAKING CHILDBIRTH CLASSES

When choosing a childbirth class, bear in mind that all childbirth educators are not the same but vary in their approach just as much as do caregivers.

A childbirth class should be small (ten couples or less) to promote group discussion. Classes should inspire confidence in both partners—in the mother's ability to birth naturally and in the father's ability to give effective labor support as he shares the childbearing miracle. Good childbirth classes will also acquaint you with your options and present home, childbearing center, and hospital birth on the same footing; support breastfeeding; and teach something about cesarean prevention, not just about cesarean surgery. If you want to birth naturally, you would do best to avoid a childbirth class that does not meet this description.

Holistic childbirth classes—those that emphasize the role of the mind and emotions, as well as the body, during childbearing—are becoming more common.

The best classes are usually taught by independent childbirth educators in private homes or on other neutral ground. Avoid classes sponsored by an institution where you plan to give birth or taught by a childbirth educator associated with your caregiver. They are rarely consumer-oriented, though there are of course exceptions.

Many childbirth educators who teach in hospitals feel unable to tell the truth about electronic fetal monitoring and other medical intervention, cesarean prevention, the parents' right to choose among various options, and so forth, for fear of losing their jobs. Many do not know the truth about these issues themselves. Though a few excellent childbirth classes are taught in hospitals, many are designed simply to create compliant patients rather than help parents achieve their individual goals. It is far better to educate yourself than to take such a class.

IF YOU ARE EXPECTING TWINS

If you are expecting twins, or triplets for that matter, you can still give birth vaginally unless there is a problem during the pregnancy or labor. Like many obstetrical situations, it is a matter of finding a caregiver who supports your goal.

IF YOU ARE TOLD YOU MUST GIVE BIRTH BY CESAREAN SECTION

Many mothers have heard that they must have a cesarean section as a result of some medical complication—anything from uterine fibroids to a prior cesarean. In some unusual circumstances such as full placenta previa (see Chapter Two), a cesarean section is the only safe way to deliver the baby. However, more often than not, the mother who is told she must have a cesarean *can* birth normally.

If you are told a cesarean section is inevitable, seek another opinion. Major abdominal surgery is not something to be accepted lightly. When you do go for another opinion, be sure the person you consult has a low cesarean rate.

If you are unable to find a caregiver willing to assist you in a vaginal birth, contact the Cesarean Prevention Movement (CPM) or C/SEC (see the Resources section at the end of this book).

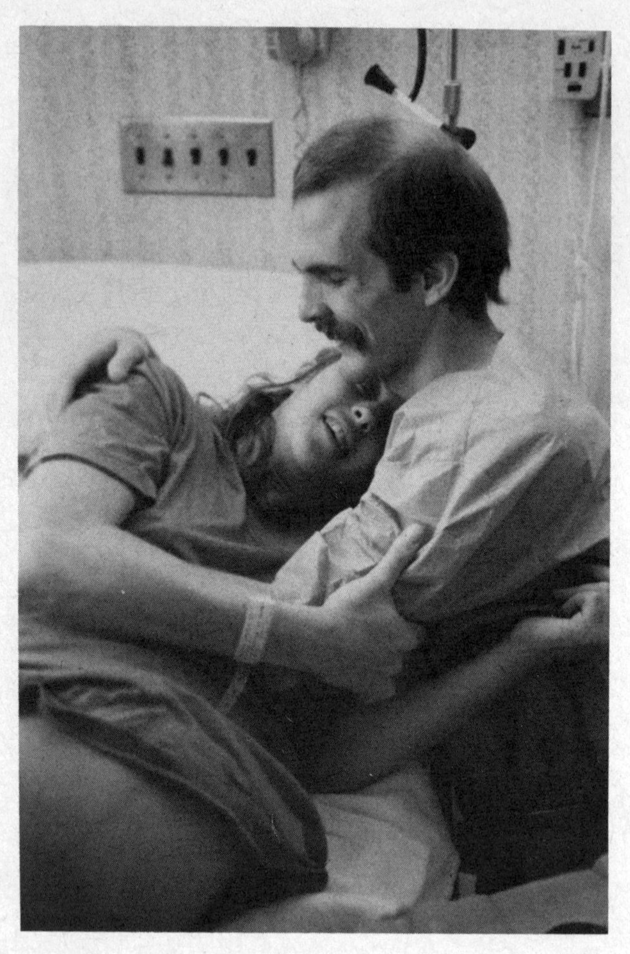

chapter five

Cesarean Prevention: Labor

Labor begins. The moment you have prepared for and awaited for nine months. Many parents ask themselves: Can this really be it? For most, labor's beginning is a time of tremendous excitement. "It was the middle of the night and contractions were thirty minutes apart and very mild," recalls Judy about her first labor. "But there was no way I could sleep. I was so excited!"

Every mother's labor is somewhat different, like every plant, every tree. There are a million variations on this exquisite theme. Some mothers labor and give birth within three or four hours, while others take a day and a night. A few have contractions on and off for several days. On the other hand, my wife, Jan, had what seemed like several days of contractions all packed into a few hours. In cases like this, the longer labor is not always the harder.

There are averages—such as the estimate that first-stage labor lasts 12½ hours and second-stage one to four hours with the first baby. But these are only averages. Every labor is unique. No one pattern will fit all.

Once labor has begun, nature will almost always work on her own without external help. There are no rules to follow, nothing you need to do but let the childbearing miracle unfold.

Meanwhile, the steps in this chapter will help you stay comfortable as they decrease your chance of surgical birth.

THE ESSENTIAL STEPS TO PREVENTING A CESAREAN DURING LABOR

During pregnancy, you and your partner should *both* get familiar with the steps in this chapter. The most important, such as having continual effective labor support, work best only if you have made careful preparations well in advance of labor.

Many of the essential steps ahead, such as laboring in the position in which you are most comfortable and eating and drinking to satisfy appetite, may seem like common sense. But since some childbirth customs in America are far removed from common sense (like depriving a laboring mother of liquids and food), the expectant parents need to be reminded of this information.

As with the cesarean-prevention measures in the last chapter, the steps here will prove most effective if you follow every single one. This is especially important if you plan a birth outside your home. In this situation, your labor is already somewhat compromised by the unfamiliar environment and your risk of cesarean increased.

Leave home for your birth place at an appropriate time. As a general rule, the mother planning a hospital birth should remain at home until contractions are intense, lasting at least forty to fifty seconds and coming every five minutes or less. By so doing, she avoids being in the hospital environment longer than necessary.

Some hospitals have more or less arbitrary deadlines regarding the length of labor. For example, the mother is perhaps expected to labor and give birth within twenty-four hours. If she does not, her labor is augmented with Pitocin. However, normal labor often lasts much longer. Some women have on-and-off contractions for several days. Remaining in the hospital environment for a prolonged period can put the mother at high risk of surgical birth. Besides, no one wants to spend several days in a hospital labor room!

On the other hand, many women would prefer to be in the place where they are going to give birth as soon as they know they are in labor. This way, the mother can settle into her environment.

Let common sense and intuition guide you. If you are giving birth in a clinical environment where a deadline is likely to be set on the length of your labor, it is obviously better to stay home until labor is active. If, however, your birth place is one where you are comfortable and you know you will be able to labor naturally as long as you please, you might prefer to leave home during early labor.

Bring your own gown to the birthing place. After all, labor is one of the biggest events of your life, and you probably will want to wear clothing that makes you feel comfortable psychologically as well as physically.

Of course, what you wear is a matter of personal preference. Some feel inhibited in a hospital gown—clothing associated with illness. Others would prefer the hospital gown to get messy rather than their own. Personally, I believe that every step you take, however minor, to remind yourself that you are radiantly healthy and at the peak of your creative power (not an invalid) is a step away from surgical birth.

Whatever you decide, be sure to keep your own clothes nearby in case your labor slows down and you want to leave the maternity area, go out for a walk, or go home.

Many women prefer to be nude, especially as labor progresses. As already stated, the mother's inhibitions are decreased as labor moves along. She is frequently unconcerned about who sees her naked body or hears the sounds she might make. It is common to see a woman remove all her clothing in a childbearing center or at home. Sometimes her partner joins her and removes his own clothing so he can hold her during labor, and later hold the baby skin to skin. This often creates a particularly sensual and beautiful childbearing scene.

Draping the mother's legs during the second stage—a common practice in some hospitals—is unnecessary. Childbearing is not a sterile procedure. Draping is largely a matter of convention, especially when the delivery room is used.

Take warm showers and baths as comfortable. Showering keeps you vertical, an especially good position for a faster labor. It also helps you relax and eases discomfort. Let the shower fall on your back or on your rolling belly.

Your partner should remain nearby—or shower with you—to help you during contractions. If he prefers, he can bring swim trunks to the hospital or childbearing center.

Most laboring mothers find baths quite relaxing and soothing. If you are in active labor, you can bathe whether or not the membranes have ruptured. Some women enjoy the bath so much that they give birth right in the tub.

Drink to satisfy thirst, and eat lightly to satisfy hunger. Though this is blatantly obvious advice, the parents should bear in mind that in some hospitals food and liquids by mouth are withheld from laboring women. This policy was originally instituted at a time when a high percentage of mothers gave birth under general anesthesia, with the risk of the mother vomiting while unconscious and asphyxiating on her stomach's contents. However, today few receive general anesthesia, and those who do are intubated to prevent aspirating regurgitated stomach contents. Yet the policy lingers.

In some hospitals, ice chips are offered laboring mothers to quench thirst. Though ice chips are often welcome, especially if the mother is sweaty, they are hardly a satisfying alternative to nourishing liquids and a hot meal.

Labor is hard work. You need nourishment, especially if your labor is long. The IV supplies energy but is no substitute for eating and drinking normally. Besides, the IV is to be avoided by anyone planning a normal birth.

As in everything in childbearing, let your body be your guide. Digestion may slow during labor but doesn't stop altogether. Most women enjoy hot tea with honey, or fruit juice. It is best to eat lightly—gelatin, hot soup, toast with jam, and so forth.

Urinate at least once every two hours. This may sound like silly advice. However, during late labor, with pressure on the bladder, you may not feel the need to urinate. Meanwhile, a full bladder can impede labor's progress. During labor, your partner should remind you to urinate.

Prepare to have continuous, effective labor support. Nothing helps a woman cope with labor as much as effective labor support. Nothing is so important if you want to prevent an unnecessary cesarean.

The support person brings out the laboring mother's inner strength by encouraging her when her spirits are failing, by cuddling and caressing her when she needs to be held, and by blanketing her with his nurturing presence.

Anyone can learn to give effective support, but no one can do this better than the father. As he shares the life-altering childbearing drama, he can reduce the pain, the fear, and in some cases even the length of his partner's labor.

Of course, the father is bound to be anxious during the birth of his own child. He, too, is experiencing labor. Yet he can still provide effective support if he has prepared for his role during pregnancy, wants to be actively involved, and is committed to helping his partner birth naturally.

It is vital for the father to learn how he can best support his partner well in advance of labor. One of my previous books, *Sharing Birth: A Father's Guide to Giving Support During Labor,* shows him precisely how to reduce his partner's fear and pain through the phases and stages of labor. The book includes methods that anyone—father, friend or childbirth professional—can use to help a woman through labor. A more concise summary of labor support methods is "The Labor Support Guide—For Fathers, Family and Friends." (See Suggested Reading.)

The essentials of effectively helping a woman through labor are: being nurturing; giving emotional support; giving encouragement; helping the mother relax; maintaining close physical contact; massaging to aid relaxation and reduce pain; and simply being there to share the experience with her. If the mother has electronic fetal monitoring, the father should avoid allowing the machines to monopolize his attention. This detracts from his ability to give effective support. Caressing, cuddling, and being spoken to in a low voice often help a woman surrender to the inner event of labor. The birthing environment should be an atmosphere in which the couple can be uninhibited and feel free to express their most intimate feelings.

Instructing the mother through breathing patterns—the major subject of many childbirth classes—is actually the father's least important activity. He can aid his partner with rhythmic breathing if she finds this helpful. But many do not. They prefer to use mental imagery or simply to relax, surrendering to each contraction. Often it is far more effective for the father simply to say "Open, open, open" in a soft voice or guide the mother through mental imagery such as "The Opening Flower" (as discussed later in this chapter).

What helps one woman may not help another. The mother must find her own way of coping with labor. This is why it is especially important for the father to be flexible. As labor unfolds, he should adjust his support method to whatever his partner finds most helpful—guided mental imagery, rhythmic breathing, or just being caressed.

Don't depend on childbirth classes to learn about labor support. Many cast the father in the role of "coach." However, the father should avoid seeing himself in this light. He is not a coach but his partner's lover, there to share a miracle—the birth of their child. Furthermore, so-called "coaching" is not an appropriate way to aid the sensitive laboring woman. The mother doesn't need instructions (though these may help at times) but nurturing, loving support.

The father, too, may need support so that he can better support his partner. If the couple chooses to hire an additional support person, they should be sure it is someone who will support them both and complement the father's role.

The father may adopt a protective role when his partner becomes so sensitive and vulnerable during labor. It is natural for him to assume this role and one of the reasons he is the ideal support person. He can interface with the staff and answer questions for his partner. In addition, he can act as a liaison, fending off unwanted medical procedures. However, as already stated, it is always best to plan your birth so that such interaction is unnecessary.

Family and Friends at Birth

"My husband, Joe, massaged my back through the entire labor and shared the experience with me," recalls Phillippa about her vaginal birth after a previous cesarean. "I didn't feel that I was doing it all myself. I felt as if we were both giving birth. In addition, my mother, aunt, and four-year-old daughter were also there. It meant a lot to us knowing that people we loved shared the experience."

Throughout history in various societies the world over, women have birthed in the presence of loved ones. Familiar, caring, understanding relatives and friends can be a tremendous help.

Some couples invite their family and/or friends to share their birth. Others prefer to be alone. If you do invite someone to be with you, be sure that whoever you choose has a positive attitude about birth.

Anyone planning to attend a birth should become familiar with the labor process and the way laboring women often behave.

It is surprising how many big and little tasks there are

when a woman is in labor: replenishing hot compresses, making hot tea and light meals, back-rubbing, taking photographs, and so on. Even children can give invaluable help, as well as a special dimension to the already wondrous childbearing miracle.

In this society, some deem it more acceptable to have strangers at a birth (such as hospital staff persons) than familiar faces—yet another one of America's perplexing childbearing customs. Find out how hospital staff persons feel about additional support persons or guests. Some are antagonistic. Some hospitals don't even permit the presence of anyone besides the father. However, any hospital that does not welcome the guests of your choice at your own birth (including a trained labor-support person, discussed ahead) is not a good environment in which to have a baby.

The Trained Labor-Support Person

Many couples today hire a trained labor-support person, often called a monitrice, doula, labor coach, childbirth assistant, or simply a support person. These persons are usually childbirth educators, midwives-in-training, or mothers who have had natural births and want to help other women.

Some childbirth educators insist that the support person must be a woman. But this, like the bias regarding the caregiver discussed in Chapter Four, is a matter of sexual prejudice. Anyone—male or female—who is sensitive, nurturing, and willing to share the experience, can help a woman through labor. "Whether a support person is male or female makes no difference," states Elisabeth Bing, one of the founders of ASPO/Lamaze, childbirth educator, and author of *Making Love During Pregnancy.* "A man can give labor support just as well as a woman."

A good support person can help the childbearing woman or couple in many ways: acting as a consumer advocate in the hospital; giving an expert opinion about any number of issues relating to the mother's labor (some do vaginal exams and help a couple decide when to go to the hospital); and complementing the father's role. He or she may give active help throughout labor or may at times remain silent in the background and help only when and if needed.

An experienced support person can be especially beneficial to couples who must give birth in a highly clinical atmosphere or who need consumer advocacy, and to mothers whose partners are unable to participate.

Some childbirth educators, however, urge all couples to hire a trained support person. They believe that the inexperienced father is unable to provide adequate support to his partner without help. A few books reflect this misconceived notion. One well-known childbirth educator recommends that all her students hire a professional to help them through labor, claiming the father doesn't know enough to give good support. Yet she spends not one single moment of her class preparing the father (and this is in the name of a holistic approach to childbirth!).

It is unfortunate that some childbirth classes so devalue the father's all-important support-giving role at a time when everything possible should be done to make him feel more confident. Good classes inspire confidence in *both* partners—the mother in her strength to birth naturally, and the father in his ability to provide effective support.

Like caregivers, labor-support persons differ in their approach. Some are simply "coaches" who instruct women with rigid breathing patterns. Others help the mother find her own way to cope best with labor.

If you plan to hire a support person, keep the following guidelines in mind:

- Meet the labor-support person in advance of your due date and discuss your birth plans. Be sure he is wholly supportive of your plans.
- Hire a support person unaffiliated with the institution where you will be laboring and unaffiliated with your caregiver. The person you choose to attend your birth should be there solely to meet your needs.
- Be sure you and your partner are both comfortable with the labor-support person.

Walk around as much as possible. Take a walk outside if you wish. If you are in active labor and prefer to remain in the hospital or childbearing center, walk around the room or the halls. Walking decreases discomfort and speeds up labor. It is also an effective way to get labor going if it has stopped or slowed down.

Once labor is active, your partner should accompany you when you walk. During contractions, you can lean on him or lean against a wall while he massages your back.

There are no rules about how often you should walk around. Let your body be your guide. If you would rather remain reclining or sitting, and your labor is active, by all means do so. My wife, Jan, spent almost the whole of her active labor virtually motionless on her side in bed because this was where she was most comfortable. Her contractions were so fast and furious that standing up and walking was nearly impossible, and she did so only when necessary to visit the bathroom. Other mothers will prefer standing up and walking around, showering, and so on, right through labor.

Adopt the position that is most comfortable for you and change position as desired.

First stage: If the mother follows her own intuition, she will almost invariably adopt the best labor and birth position for her. Generally speaking, upright positions such as standing, sitting, kneeling on all fours, and walking are best for first-stage labor. Several studies have shown that the vertical position decreases discomfort, increases the speed of labor, and may even decrease the incidence of fetal distress.[1]

Avoid lying flat on your back. This can cause maternal hypotension (low blood pressure) as a result of pressure from the heavy uterus on the inferior vena cava and reduce the amount of oxygen reaching your baby, causing fetal distress. The supine (back-lying) position can also lead to less-efficient and more painful uterine contractions as well as a longer labor.

You should have freedom of movement throughout labor and never be restricted from changing positions or moving about as you wish. This is another good reason to avoid intravenous feeding and electronic fetal monitoring. If you must have an IV, request that it be on a mobile stand. If EFM is used, it should be alternated with periods of walking about. Restricted mobility can impair labor's progress and lead to fetal distress, with a resultant cesarean.

Second stage: As with first-stage labor, the second stage is often easier if the mother is in a vertical position. Other positions for second stage are:

- Lying on the side. A good position if you are tired.
- Semi-reclining, head and shoulders well supported by pillows. Though not the ideal position for an efficient

labor, for many mothers it is the most comfortable.

• Squatting on bed or floor with partner's support. You can sit up or go forward to a hands-and-knees position between contractions if you find prolonged squatting uncomfortable (as do most American women). The birth canal is slightly shortened, and the pelvic outlet is expanded by an average of 28 percent in the squatting, as compared to the supine, position.[2] In addition, gravity is on your side. Squatting can shorten an otherwise long bearing-down stage and is especially helpful if the baby is in a posterior position.

• Sitting on a toilet or birthing chair. (For many, this is the most comfortable birthing position.)

• On hands and knees (put a pillow or mat under the knees for comfort).

• Standing leaning against a wall or against your partner.

The recumbent position is a matter of custom that evolved solely for the convenience of the caregiver. If your caregiver is inexperienced in delivering babies in any other position (as are many physicians and midwives), simply adopt the position you prefer until birth is imminent. Then switch at your caregiver's direction.

Let your body be your guide about when and how to push. It is almost always better to wait until you feel the urge to push before you bear down, even if you are fully dilated. Occasionally, the mother reaches full dilation and needs a rest before the urge to give birth sweeps over her (though more often she feels like pushing right away).

Avoid prolonged breath-holding during bearing down (this can lead to fetal distress).

Avoid stirrups. Legs in stirrups during second stage makes pushing more difficult and increases your chance of tearing, an episiotomy, and forceps delivery. Stirrups may be useful for certain gynecological procedures and perhaps for the repair of lacerations and use of forceps when truly necessary. However, when it comes to childbirth, this is another of those customs best avoided.

Avoid time limits. Your labor may be much longer or shorter than average and still be perfectly normal. Let it unfold in its own individual way unless there is a genuine medical complication. Be sure your caregiver supports this way of handling your labor.

Express yourself freely and without inhibition. Many women find vocal expression one of the best aids to coping with labor. Moaning, sighing, and groaning can all relieve tension and are often the childbearing woman's natural way of expressing herself. As already stated, the laboring mother frequently sounds like a woman at the height of sexual passion. The sensual sounds she makes and her uninhibited behavior are part of her primitive beauty. On the other hand, you may make sounds that have little resemblance to the sounds of lovemaking. This is also fine. "I sounded about as sexy as a cow, bellowing my way through late first stage," one mother said.

Your partner should understand how laboring women often sound and encourage free expression.

If you find yourself on the verge of panic during late labor, when contractions may be particularly difficult, try lowering the pitch of your voice and groaning. This is often an effective way to dissolve fear. Your partner can remind you to do this if the need arises.

Use mental imagery to help you relax and cope with labor. According to Suzanna May Hilbers, teacher trainer for ASPO/Lamaze, this is the most powerful method there is of reducing the fear and pain of labor. She states: "Mental imagery can actually bring about physiological changes and alter the course of labor."[3]

As the inner event of labor (discussed in Chapter Four) unfolds, the mother enters an altered mind state during which she is particularly open to the power of mental imagery. Using imagery can help you surrender to the childbearing process, thereby creating a more efficient labor. In addition, it may even help speed cervical dilation in ways that we don't yet understand.

The following three exercises are from the book *Mind Over Labor.*[4] Many additional exercises are included in that book. You can do these exercises yourself or your partner can guide you through them by sitting nearby and speaking in a soft voice. For best results, he should practice the imagery exercises with you during pregnancy.

The Opening Flower

Many laboring women find this simple imagery quite effective. There is no better analogue for the dilating cervix during first stage and the stretching birth canal during second stage than the blossoming flower, an image that combines warmth, moisture, and beauty with the idea of opening.

Use this imagery any time during labor. You can also use it if labor stops or slows down.

Marian Tompson, co-founder of La Leche League International and co-author of the bestselling *The Womanly Art of Breastfeeding,* used this very exercise during her daughter Allison's labor. An avid supporter of natural birth,

Marian Tompson helped all her five daughters through labor while enjoying the supreme pleasure of attending her grandchildren's births. Coincidentally, on the day Allison went into labor, Ms. Tompson received in the mail the manuscript of *Mind Over Labor,* for which she planned to write a foreword. She brought the manuscript with her to Allison's house. After twenty-four hours of labor, Allison's contractions slowed down. They tried everything to get it going. Finally, Marian Tompson decided to guide her through "The Opening Flower" as suggested in the manuscript. Shortly afterward, Allison's contractions picked up. According to Ms. Tompson, using imagery at that time, along with the continuous support of her husband and a reassuring caregiver, gave Allison what she needed to carry on superbly.

> Imagine a beautiful flower. Choose any flower you want—a rose, a lily, even the thousand-petaled lotus so often figured in Oriental imagery—as long as it is beautiful to you.
>
> Imagine that it is gradually expanding, petal by petal, until it is fully opened.
>
> You can add as much detail as you want—dew on the petals, warm sun rays, fragrance, and so forth. You can even picture or sense yourself standing in a garden surrounded by hundreds of flowers and imagine that you have chosen this one special opening flower to observe.

Imagining the Birth

Many women find that imagining the physical details of the birth helps labor to progress more smoothly. Don't be concerned whether or not your mental picture of the cervix dilating or the baby descending in the birth canal is accurate. Often, mental imagery speaks in the language of metaphor (like "The Opening Flower"), and your mind will make the connection.

Imagine yourself opening. Envision the baby's head against the cervix and the cervix widening to let it pass.

At the same time, mentally say "yes" to the contractions as they come and fade away.

Remind yourself that the more powerful contractions are the most effective. They massage and stimulate the baby as they open the birth passage and push the baby downward.

With each contraction, imagine the baby moving through the birth passage, closer and closer to your waiting arms.

The Special Place

You can use this imagery at any time during pregnancy or labor. It is a very effective aid to relaxation.

Practice "The Special Place" during pregnancy. Share the details of your special place with your partner. This way, when you are in labor, he can help you relax by recalling some of the images you have chosen.

Get in a comfortable position and relax.

Breathe deeply and rhythmically.

Imagine each breath you take in as bringing health-giving life energy and each breath you let out carrying tension away.

Continue breathing this way for a minute or so, and feel yourself entering a more peaceful relaxed state of mind and body.

Now imagine that you are in a special place that is peaceful and makes you feel secure and comfortable. It can be any place at all, real or imaginary: a favorite room, a beautiful natural setting—a meadow, a bubbling brook, the ocean—anywhere you feel completely safe and comfortable.

Let the details of this special place unfold.

Acknowledge that this is your own place. No one can enter without your invitation.

Take a few minutes to explore this place and enjoy it. You can return here at any time and feel peaceful and completely relaxed.

Avoid pain medication. All obstetrical analgesia and anesthesia affect uterine contractions, and can impair labor. Frequently, the use of pain medication breeds more intervention. For example, drugs can slow labor down, causing the caregiver to initiate hormonal augmentation (see page 113), which may in turn precipitate the need for a cesarean. In addition, no medication has proven entirely safe for the baby.

Of course, the final choice about pain medication must remain yours. Only you know what you are feeling and whether or not it is needed. However, under most circumstances medication can be avoided.

The most important factors in avoiding pain medication are:

1. the strong desire to birth naturally;
2. the continuous support of your partner and/or other labor-support person;
3. an obstetrical staff that supports natural birth;
4. the use of nonpharmacologic pain-relief methods.

Be sure your partner supports you in your resolve to avoid drugs. Mothers frequently ask for medication toward the end of first stage when labor is most difficult. At this time, what the laboring woman most often needs is her partner's reassurance and his effective labor support. Through massage, relaxation, guided mental imagery, and so forth, in most cases the father can help the mother cope with labor naturally.

Avoid all medical intervention unless there is a complication. This includes intravenous feeding and continuous electronic fetal monitoring. All medical intervention interferes with the normal labor process. (See Chapter Three.)

Avoid hormonal labor induction or augmentation. If labor does not progress, some caregivers prescribe intravenous Pitocin to augment contractions. This is frequently the first step on the road to a cesarean. As discussed in Chapter Three, Pitocin usually causes more painful contractions, which come on suddenly and are more difficult to manage. There is therefore a greater need for medication, which can impair labor, leading to the use of more Pitocin and so on. In addition, Pitocin-induced contractions often lead to fetal distress, one of the prime indications for cesarean birth.

See the sections on "If Your Labor Is Overdue" and "If Your Labor Stops or Slows Down" (later in this chapter) for safe alternatives to Pitocin.

Avoid excessive vaginal exams during labor. Numerous exams are commonly done in large hospitals where the laboring woman is attended by several nurses and residents as well as her caregiver. However, too many vaginal exams can be uncomfortable and increase your chance of infection.

Feel free to refuse any routine medical procedure that you do not wish. Sometimes, emergencies arise and medical intervention is necessary for the well-being of mother and baby. But this doesn't mean you should have to submit to routine procedures if there is no medical problem.

Bear in mind that it is your birth, your baby. You, not your caregiver or the hospital staff, are the center of the childbearing drama. Think of your caregiver and the staff as your hired help.

You will no doubt feel dependent, vulnerable, and highly sensitive during labor and hardly feel like asserting your rights. Let your partner be your spokesperson. For example, if a nurse offers pain-relief medication, he can say, "We've discussed this together prior to labor and my wife has decided to labor without medication." Of course, if he says this he must be sure that he is actually expressing your wishes.

If you must refuse a particular procedure such as an IV, do so as politely as possible. But be firm. You or your partner can say, "We have researched the matter and do not choose to have an IV unless absolutely necessary in the event of a medical problem."

You may have to sign a waiver if you refuse a routine procedure. This is common at most hospitals.

Though you have the right to refuse any unwanted procedure, it is always preferable to choose a suitable birth place and caregiver so that insisting upon your rights is unnecessary. During labor, you should feel able to let go and be wholly open—not feel as if you were going to battle.

IF YOUR MEMBRANES RUPTURE PRIOR TO LABOR

When membranes rupture spontaneously, water is discharged in a trickle or a gush. This is frequently a sign that labor will begin, usually within six to forty-eight hours.

If your labor does not begin spontaneously within this time, you are at greater risk of infection. However, this by no means implies that you must give birth within twenty-four to forty-eight hours, as some caregivers and hospitals insist. If the mother with ruptured membranes is not in active labor at the end of twenty-four hours or so (the time varies with different caregivers), some physicians induce labor or even perform a cesarean.

Generally speaking, there is no reason for you to be in a hospital and have your labor augmented when membranes rupture. Usually, the best place to be is at home, where you are not at high risk of a cesarean. In some cases, the membranes may reseal. However, you should take certain precautions if membranes rupture:

- Consult your caregiver to be sure the baby's head is engaged (deep in the bony pelvis) to rule out the possibility of cord prolapse (a grave complication).
- Avoid tub baths until you are in active labor, at which time tub baths may prove relaxing.
- Avoid intercourse.
- Don't put anything, including a tampon, into the vagina.
- Take your temperature regularly. If it rises, consult your caregiver without delay.
- Drink plenty of fluids, including fruit juice.

If your caregiver insists on aggressive management of labor (and there are no medical complications), consult another caregiver who knows how to handle every ROM in a more natural manner. See the NAPSAC *Directory of Alternative Birth Services* (see Resources). Consulting another caregiver at this late date may be extremely inconvenient, but it is far less so than having a cesarean.

IF YOUR LABOR IS OVERDUE

Labor begins right on the due date only about 5 percent of the time. Pregnancy lasts approximately 266 days from the date of conception, or 280 days (ten lunar months of twenty-eight days each) from the first day of your last menstrual period. The due date is usually estimated by subtracting three calendar months from the first day of your last menstrual period and then adding seven days. There are several reasons why your due date is only an estimate: (1) The length of human gestation varies. (2) The length of the menstrual cycle varies, and it is not always possible to determine the date of conception. A mother with a menstrual cycle of thirty-two days will have a conception date several days later than the mother with a twenty-five day cycle. (3) Calendar months vary in length. However, birth usually takes place within two weeks before or after the due date.

If labor is slightly overdue, there is usually no cause for concern. However, if labor is more than two or three weeks late, and your caregiver is concerned, it might be best to consider labor induction.

The two most common medical means of inducing labor are artificial rupture of the membranes (ROM) and intravenous use of Pitocin.

As already stated, ROM increases the chance of a cesarean by setting the clock in motion and possibly causing fetal distress. The use of Pitocin carries several risks, discussed in Chapter Three. Unless there is a medical emergency, natural means of inducing labor should be tried first.

The following will work only if the cervix is *ripe* (softened, partially effaced, and sometimes partially dilated), and you are ready to go into labor. They are all quite safe. However, do consult your caregiver before trying them to be sure there are no medical contraindications.

- Take a long walk (two to four miles), preferably up and down hills.

- Take a hot shower or bath and relax.
- Eat spicy, gas-producing food. The increased intestinal activity often triggers the uterus into belated action.
- Make love vigorously and with orgasm if possible (no intercourse if membranes have ruptured). This releases the hormone oxytocin, which, combined with the effects of physical activity, may initiate labor. Oral or manual nipple stimulation will also release oxytocin and may initiate contractions.
- Discuss with your partner (or a childbirth counselor) any concerns or fears you may have about birth or becoming a mother. Emotions can be the cause of an overdue labor.
- Try mental imagery. "The Opening Flower" and "Imagining the Birth" exercises may be effective.
- Give yourself an enema. Since this is the least-pleasant method, you may want to use it only if all else fails.
- Some midwives and physicians recommend castor oil induction (according to Elizabeth Davis in *A Guide to Midwifery*): Take 2 tablespoons by mouth, followed by 1 tablespoon in one half hour, with a repeat dose in another half hour.

IF YOUR LABOR STOPS OR SLOWS DOWN

A labor that has stopped or slowed down is not necessarily abnormal. A few mothers have on-and-off contractions for several days before their labor becomes active. This is simply the way childbearing is for some women. Patience on the part of both parents is essential. Meanwhile, one of the most important factors in the management of this type of labor is a caregiver willing to let labor unfold naturally.

Medical intervention should be used *only* if necessary. Using drugs to augment a labor that has slowed down is often a case of repairing something that's already working, only to have it really break down.

False Labor

Many mothers have checked into the hospital or childbearing center only to discover that they were not really in labor. This is quite common. Women often have contractions that are not part of real labor.

To distinguish false from true labor, bear in mind that false labor contractions: (1) usually occur at irregular intervals; (2) don't become stronger as time passes; (3) often stop or slow down with a change of activity; (4) may stop after an alcoholic drink; (5) are not accompanied by other signs of labor; and (6) do not dilate the cervix.

Sometimes, true labor that has been active takes a pause, like a hiker stopping for a rest midway up the mountain. This doesn't mean that labor is petering out or somehow abnormal. It may just be the way your labor is unfolding.

Occasionally, the cause of a stopped labor is physical. However, emotional factors can and often do cause labor to slow down or stop entirely. Several studies have shown that disturbance in the birthing environment impairs labor and even affects the outcome of the offspring.[5] Other factors that can prolong labor and perhaps lead to fetal distress and a resultant cesarean include tension between you and your partner; the presence of someone with whom you are uncomfortable; inhibitions; and strong negative feelings about becoming a mother. Handling a prolonged labor is often a matter of dealing with the emotional factors responsible.

Ideally, your caregiver should convey that everything is

fine. However, when labor takes longer than average, few actually radiate this confidence. For this reason, it is important for *you* to know that a pause in labor may be perfectly natural.

Arrange to be alone with your partner for a while. Everyone knows that a watched pot doesn't boil. When someone is standing by waiting for labor to become active, the mother often becomes anxious, wondering if her body is indeed performing correctly. The very pressure to "perform" impairs labor.

Unless there is a medical emergency, try natural means of augmenting labor before resorting to Pitocin, which, as already stated in Chapter Three, carries several risks and markedly increases your chance of a cesarean.

All the methods discussed ahead are safe. However, check with your caregiver to be sure there are no contraindications in your case.

Early Labor

If early labor (cervix dilated less than four centimeters) stops or slows down, more often than not the best thing to do is forget about it. As long as the baby is fine, you don't need to do anything. Just go about your daily life and labor will most likely resume later on.

Women often have a long period of uterine contractions that don't necessarily dilate the cervix. This is referred to as *prodromal* labor and may last anywhere from a few minutes to several days. Certified nurse midwife Fran Ventre compares prodromal labor to "the time the orchestra spends tuning up. They are playing their instruments and making noise, but they have not started the piece yet. At some point the conductor raises the baton and they begin to play the music. The tuning up time is necessary, however, and some take longer to tune up than others."[6]

For some mothers, prodromal contractions can be painful and frustrating, especially if they seem to go on endlessly.

If contractions are persistent yet not dilating the cervix, you may have difficulty going about your daily life or sleeping. In this case, there are several things to try:

- Relax.
- Get your mind off labor. Sometimes this is all that is needed. Watch TV, visit with friends, take a walk, take a hot bath or shower, have a glass of wine, and so forth.
- Change your environment. If you are in a hospital and in early labor, by all means consider going home or for a walk outdoors. Spending several hours or days in the same labor room "waiting for it to happen" is enough to drive anyone to surgical delivery.

Active Labor

Active labor (cervix more than four to five centimeters dilated) often stops or slows down shortly after admission to the hospital. Presumably, the cause is anxiety at being moved to an unfamiliar environment. Considering the sensitive inner event of labor, one might expect such a reaction. On the other hand, sometimes labor will not become active until a mother reaches the hospital or birthing center. This is probably because she feels safest there and unconsciously holds back her labor until she is in the birth place of her choice.

Often when active labor slows down, it picks up a little later on its own. However, if labor does not get going again, try the steps ahead. Meanwhile, be sure to drink sweet liquids such as tea with honey, and fruit juice to restore your energy and body fluids.

- Rest or sleep if possible.
- Relaxation.
- A warm shower or bath.
- A change of position. Squatting and pelvic rocking on all fours are helpful if the baby's head is in the posterior position (back of the skull against the mother's spine).
- Walking.
- Lovemaking. This causes the release of the hormone oxytocin and may intensify contractions (no intercourse if membranes have ruptured).
- Nipple stimulation. This also causes oxytocin to be released. You can stimulate your nipples manually or have your partner do it.
- If someone in the environment is making you uncomfortable, ask that person to leave for a while.
- If there is tension between you and your partner at this particularly anxious time of life, try to work it out.
- If you are uncomfortable in the environment and there is nothing you can do about it, try turning down the lights, playing soft music, using mental imagery, and paying special attention to labor support.
- If you feel the cause is emotional, talk over any concerns you may have about becoming a mother or about birth.
- Use mental imagery. Effective imagery exercises for a flagging labor include "The Special Place" and "The Opening Flower." In addition, you can imagine the cervix opening a gateway for your baby. Imagine the baby descending, down through the birth canal, and finally emerging to your waiting arms.

If none of the above methods work, and you and your caregiver opt for Pitocin augmentation, you should take several precautions to minimize your chances of surgical birth. Pitocin-induced or -augmented contractions are often more difficult to manage than natural labor contractions. They tend to rise suddenly to a peak and to be more intense. Request that the dose be the minimum needed to regulate contractions. Meanwhile, your partner's support is especially important. He should be at your side constantly, helping you relax and using all the nonpharmacological means he can to relieve pain.

Second Stage

After the cervix is fully dilated, birth usually takes place within twenty minutes to three hours. However, some mothers have a longer second stage. Though exhausting, an extended second stage is not abnormal as long as there are no signs of fetal distress.

You can help a long or difficult second stage progress by changing positions to make yourself comfortable. Adopt vertical positions: squatting with your partner's support; sitting on a birthing chair or toilet; standing and leaning against the wall or your partner.

Push only with your body's urge. Avoid holding your breath while pushing.

Above all, don't give up. One of the most important aids during a lengthy second stage is the unflagging support of your partner.

IF YOU MUST LABOR IN A CLINICAL ENVIRONMENT

The healthy mother whose pregnancy is normal should choose a nonclinical birthing environment. Unfortunately, this is not always possible for the woman with a difficult pregnancy. If, as a result of some medical problem, you must birth in a clinical setting, you can still have a normal labor and lower your chance of a cesarean. However, it will take extra effort.

Following are some things to soften the impact of the environment:

- Put special emphasis on effective labor support. This is your partner's job. He should learn everything he can about helping you through labor. His support is vital to a normal labor if you are birthing in a clinical setting.
- Consider hiring an additional labor-support person. An experienced helper can often act as a liaison between you and the obstetrical staff and help you feel as comfortable as you can in the unfamiliar setting. He or she can also complement the father's role.
- Bring a tape recorder and some cassettes of your favorite music to create your own background sounds.
- Use mental imagery. Create our own internal environment with peaceful, relaxing images. There are also several mental-imagery tapes available for use during labor (see Suggested Reading).

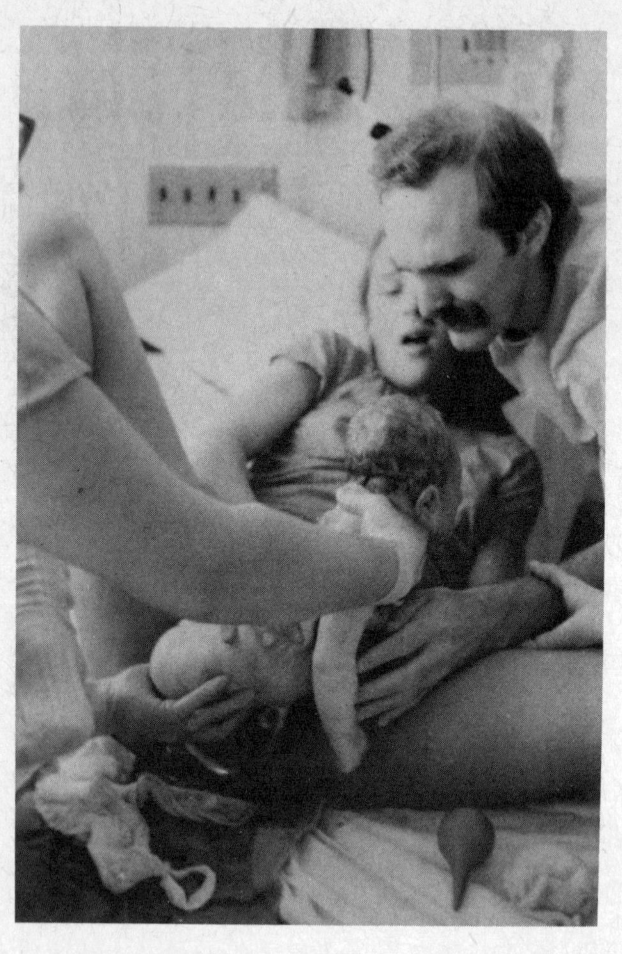

chapter six

Natural Birth After a Previous Cesarean

In 1978, 98.9 percent of mothers in the United States who had prior cesareans were delivered by repeat cesarean following subsequent pregnancies.[1] The repeat cesarean rate in many institutions is close to 100 percent.[2] This is perhaps the single most appalling childbirth statistic in American history. It is also one of the strangest. For innumerable studies have proven that *the overwhelming majority of repeat cesareans are unnecessary.*

The often-quoted seventy-year-old dictum "once a cesarean, always a cesarean" coined by the obstetrician Edward B. Craigin in 1916[3] has been disproven over and over in a multitude of medical studies. Meanwhile, repeat cesareans are responsible for 35 percent of all cesareans performed in the United States. Our overall cesarean rate would be reduced tremendously if a high percentage of mothers with previous surgical deliveries opted for and prepared for vaginal birth.

And every year, thousands of families would be far happier.

VAGINAL BIRTH AFTER CESAREAN (VBAC): THE BEST ALTERNATIVE

For decades, studies have been published in support of VBAC (a term coined in 1974 by Nancy Wainer Cohen, a leading expert and outspoken pioneer in the field of cesarean prevention). Scores of diligent researchers have discovered that vaginal birth after cesarean is far safer than repeat cesarean. It also eliminates surgical birth trauma, the effects of which are discussed in Chapter One. Meanwhile, during the last fifty years, no studies have suggested that VBAC is so dangerous that universal elective cesarean should be the rule. There aren't even any studies that discourage VBAC for healthy mothers. Even Dr. Craigin, whose "once a cesarean, always a cesarean" was to become the epitaph of natural birth for mothers with previous cesareans, admitted that there could be exceptions. Writing in 1916, he called "once a cesarean . . ." merely the usual rule, not a universal law. Moreover, he stated that *one of his own patients had given birth three times vaginally after a previous cesarean.*

According to Drs. Paul Meier and Richard Porreco, "In properly selected patients, a trial of labor after previous cesarean delivery constitutes the best and safest form of obstetric management."[4] Kaiser Foundation Hospital in San Diego, California, where these two physicians conducted revealing studies in support of VBAC, adopted a program of "trial of labor" for those who had had cesareans. The results were so overwhelmingly positive that seven Kaiser physicians suggested that patients who filled the criteria for trial of labor should not be offered the choice of elective repeat cesarean. The advantages of VBAC were too great.

Advantages of a Natural Birth After a Previous Cesarean

"There is no comparison between my third birth, a home VBAC, and my second, which was a cesarean," states Phillippa. "I felt so much more in control of my situation and my body. I had a lot more power over what was happening and how it was happening."

Jo-Ellen, whose first birth was a cesarean for a breech baby and whose second was a hospital VBAC, agrees. "The second was far less traumatic. I wasn't scared half to death of an operation—the last thing you need when you are about to become a mother. I was able to take an active part in the birth process, working with my labor rather than being a helpless, immobile invalid. Postpartum recovery was infinitely easier and far less uncomfortable. Just seeing my daughter Stacey being born, touching her head, lifting her to my abdomen, made the supreme difference. What a thrill!"

Sharon says, "I had two cesareans before I finally delivered vaginally, and the last birth was one of the most wonderful experiences I've ever had!" Her husband, Eric, shares her feelings. "I was left out in the waiting room during the first cesarean—worrying, feeling miserable. During the second cesarean, I was right there with Sharon, talking with her and still feeling anxious. During our third birth, I watched the head emerge while my eyes welled with tears. I was ecstatic!"

Following are some of the advantages of VBAC:

• *Less likelihood of postpartum illness.* According to the NIH report, postpartum fever is far less common in mothers who deliver vaginally than in those who have elective repeat cesareans.

• *Less likelihood of postpartum depression.* The incidence of postpartum depression is significantly higher among mothers who are delivered by repeat cesareans than among those who give birth vaginally.[5]

• *A much smoother, easier postpartum period.* Caring for the new baby, breastfeeding, and adjusting to motherhood are far easier after a natural vaginal birth than after an operation, when the mother is in need of medical care.

• *A safer birth for mother and baby.* According to *Cesarean Childbirth,* "Repeat cesarean carries two times the risk for maternal mortality of vaginal delivery."[6] Dr. C. J. Pauerstein compared the *best* results associated with elective repeat cesarean with the *worst* results associated with a trial of labor and came up with startling figures. The risk of maternal death associated with trial of labor was *one-fortieth* the risk associated with elective repeat cesarean, while the risk of perinatal death was *one-fourth* to *one-fifth.*[7]

• A trial of labor also eliminates the possibility of *iatrogenic* (doctor-caused) prematurity. Respiratory distress resulting from cesarean delivery, as mentioned before, is a primary cause of perinatal death. Meanwhile, babies delivered by elective cesarean often require respiratory support *even if they are not premature.*[8] One study at the University of Colorado Health Sciences Center showed that 13 percent of infants delivered by elective repeat cesarean required respiratory support, as compared to 3 percent of those delivered vaginally.[9]

• *A better beginning for the new family.* Mother, father, siblings and new baby are more likely to be happy and psychologically healthy after a normal birth.

• *Shorter or no time in the hospital.*

• *Decreased cost.* As already stated, cesarean surgery is far more expensive than vaginal birth.

For optimum results, it is best to opt for a wholly *natural* birth, not merely a VBAC. Natural birth doesn't simply mean that the baby is born vaginally. It means birth without medical intervention or drugs. Many mothers think of VBAC alone as the goal, forgetting that vaginal birth in some hospitals means laboring in a drug-induced stupor with intravenous feeding, electronic fetal monitoring, and giving birth in a highly clinical atmosphere.

Is the Incision Safe?

Various incisions are used for cesarean surgery.

There are two types of abdominal incision:

1. The *Pfannenstiel* (sometimes called the *bikini* incision) is a horizontal cut made above the pubic hairline. This is the most common type.

2. The *midline* is a vertical incision running from a little below the navel to just above the pubic hairline. This is the fastest to cut and sometimes is used in rare emergencies when speed is an issue.

The abdominal incision does not indicate the type of uterine incision. The type of *uterine* incision is what should be considered when planning a normal birth after a cesarean.

There are three types of uterine incision used for surgical birth:

1. The *low transverse* (sometimes called *low segment* or *Kerr* incision) is a horizontal incision in the lower part of the uterus near the cervix. It is the most common and most preferred method for cesarean delivery under ordinary circumstances and is used in over 90 percent of cesareans today. It has the lowest incidence of hemorrhage and the lowest incidence of rupture in subsequent pregnancies.[10]

2. The *low vertical* (or *Kroenig*) incision is used rarely, in cases of unusual presentation such as transverse lie or if the baby is very large or very small. The risk of rupture may be greater since one can't be sure how much of the uterus was incised.[11]

3. The once-common *classic incision* (a vertical incision in the upper part of the uterus) is sometimes used for unusual presentations or if the placenta covers the lower uterine segment.[12] This is the incision associated with the greatest risk among VBAC mothers. One study concluded that 90 percent of all uterine ruptures and 96 percent of perinatal deaths resulting from uterine rupture occurred among those patients with a classical incision.[13]

The type of uterine scar is included in your medical records. If you are currently visiting a new caregiver, your records should be requested as part of routine procedure.

Uterine Rupture

The major risk to the mother during vaginal birth after a previous cesarean is that of uterine rupture. The degree of risk varies directly with the type of surgical incision. True uterine rupture is occasionally associated with the classic incision but is very rare in the low transverse incision.

In fact, when it comes to a low transverse segment rupture, in the majority of cases the term "rupture" is quite misleading and what Cohen and Estner call "a despicable abuse of the English language."[14] What is referred to as a rupture is most often a *dehiscence,* a partial opening along the scar seam.

There is a world of difference between a true rupture and a dehiscence or a window. The former implies an actual separation of the entire scar for its full length. This often involves massive bleeding, rupture of the fetal membranes, and extrusion of the fetus into the abdominal cavity, resulting in the death of the baby about 50 percent of the time. (This is because most uterine ruptures occur before labor outside the hospital. The risk is far less if rupture occurs in a hospital with immediate surgical facilities available.) Dehiscence, on the other hand, refers to an often painless condition in which there is minimal or no bleeding and the fetus is not extruded into the abdominal cavity. Usually there are no complications to mother or baby as a result of scar dehiscence, and the separation need not be repaired. In fact, such a "rupture" frequently goes completely unnoticed and is self-healing. These defects are often present throughout pregnancy.

Dehiscence often occurs prior to labor's onset. The asymptomatic separation is frequently discovered while performing a repeat cesarean. According to Dr. Meier, uterine separation "occurs with equal frequency in patients who are allowed to labor or who are electively delivered by repeat cesarean."[15]

In the words of Beth Shearer, one of the nation's leading

experts on cesarean birth and a pioneer in the field of VBAC, "All the recent studies have found the incidence of scar separation to be about the same with elective cesareans as after a trial of labor."[16,17]

One reason actually cited for performing repeat cesareans is the threat of maternal death resulting from complete rupture. Obviously, everything possible should be done to avoid such a catastrophe regardless of how rare it may be. But just how frequent is death from a ruptured uterus? In the words of Dr. Justin P. Lavin, Associate Professor of Obstetrics and Gynecology at Northeastern University College of Medicine and an often-quoted expert on cesarean birth: "The English literature since 1930 does not contain a single case report of maternal death due to rupture of a low transverse uterine scar among women with a prior cesarean section undergoing trial of labor in an industrialized nation."[18]

Deaths from uterine rupture, however, have occurred in mothers who have *not* had a previous section. This is extremely rare. Yet maternal death is more common when an unscarred uterus ruptures than when rupture occurs along a scar.

What about the baby? According to Beth Shearer in *Frankly Speaking,* a handbook for cesarean couples published by C/SEC, "Over the past 30 years, only one or two infant deaths have been associated with rupture of a low transverse uterine scar, although it is not clear if the deaths were caused by the rupture or by another cause."[19]

Some say that the risk of uterine rupture is increased if there have been multiple cesarean births, multiple vaginal births following the initial cesarean, or if the placenta implants over the incision site. However, according to Dr. Lavin, there is no evidence to support this view.[20]

In one study, Dr. R. G. Douglas and his associates found that there were no emergencies as a result of rupture in 3,000 mothers who had given birth vaginally after prior cesareans.[21] In a British medical study conducted by Dr. Geoffrey A. Morewood and associates of the University Department of Obstetrics and Gynecology, St. Mary's Hospital, Manchester, England, the incidence of uterine rupture was zero and that of dehiscence 1.3 percent *without* fetal or maternal complications. Other studies show an incidence of rupture as 0.5–1.5 percent and dehiscence as 2.7–15 percent.[22]

As Dr. Morewood points out: "We must question the advisability of routine elective repeat cesarean section particularly when patients are subjected to general anesthesia, blood transfusion and increased postoperative mortality and morbidity, including wound infection, pulmonary and urinary infection, phlebitis and embolus as well as an increase in hospital stay."[23]

In fact, laboring after a previous cesarean is in most circumstances so safe that Nancy Wainer Cohen recommends home birth to healthy mothers who feel comfortable laboring in their own home. Of 173 labors she has personally followed (many of which took place at home), symptoms of uterine rupture have never been a problem.[24]

If you had a classic incision, the risks of rupture and resultant fetal death are higher (between a 1 and 3 percent risk of rupture, according to Beth Shearer.)[25] Some parents will opt for repeat cesarean. Others may choose vaginal delivery. You must weigh the risks. If you do opt for vaginal delivery, it may be best to labor and birth in a hospital rather than at home.

However, home is the only place some parents can have a vaginal birth after a classical incision. The hospitals near their home refuse care to the VBAC mother with a classical incision, insisting that she must deliver surgically. Couples in this situation often do choose a home birth. You must consider the choices and make your own decision. You may be able to find a caregiver to attend you at home. Some mothers with a classical incision have actually had to fly halfway across the country to find a birthing place and caregiver who would support their choice of vaginal birth.

In the rare circumstances when complete rupture occurs, shock may be caused from uterine hemorrhage, and a *hysterectomy* (removal of the uterus) is sometimes necessary as a result of bleeding and tissue damage.

However, most physicians who support VBAC agree that if the uterus does rupture it can usually be repaired without resorting to hysterectomy. Whether or not hysterectomy is performed depends largely on the type and extent of uterine tear and the practice of the physician. This is why it is especially important to choose your caregiver carefully and to be sure that he or she fully supports vaginal birth after cesarean.

Resistance to VBAC

During the summer of 1982, I was caught in an impossible traffic jam at one of Boston's busiest intersections. Horns honked. Frustrated drivers rammed their heads out the windows and swore. It was an endless circle of frustration. Cars going one way were waiting to turn against another line of cars waiting to turn in another direction. No one moved. Finally the driver in front of me leapt out of his car and shouted at the traffic officer who stood bewildered in the middle of the mess. "Do something about this!" he demanded.

The policeman stared at the angry man and threw his arms up into the air. "What do you want me to do?"

Countering resistance to VBAC is quite similar. It's a mess. The bewildered consumer turns to her obstetrician. Studies have proven that VBAC is safe—indeed, far safer than repeat cesarean. She demands that her obstetrician give her a chance. The obstetrician turns to the medical community. Repeat cesarean is the acceptable standard of practice. If he deviates from that, he risks a malpractice suit should anything go wrong. He points to the insurance companies, which have made it financially infeasible to practice decent obstetrics as a result of high malpractice premiums. The insurance companies point to the consumer, who might sue. Around and around and around, and it all goes nowhere.

Despite the obvious advantages of VBAC, repeat cesarean is still practically the rule in the United States. Only 6–7 percent of women who had prior cesareans had vaginal births in 1985.[26] This is not so in many other countries, including the United Kingdom, where a trial of labor is taken for granted.

Ruth, a mother who had a previous cesarean for a footling breech, moved to Israel, where she became pregnant again. "When I relayed my American gynecologist's admonitions of 'Once a cesarean, always a cesarean' and 'You don't want a ruptured uterus,' my Israeli doctor's retort came sharply: 'American doctors practice litigation, not medicine!' " Ruth's daughter Lilach was born vaginally. She gratefully recalls: "To think that had she been born in the United States, chances are that Lilach's mother would have undergone major, unnecessary surgery."[27]

There are several reasons why repeat cesareans are so common in the United States: the preference of physicians and mothers, established practice trends, and fear of malpractice suits. None of these justifies a repeat cesarean.

Since cesarean section is relatively safe, today obstetricians find it easy to opt for surgical birth. In addition, many have been taught to believe that VBAC is dangerous (though it remains a mystery why they don't learn the facts).

According to Drs. Meier and Porreco:

> Residents in obstetrics must be given adequate exposure to patients who labor after cesarean delivery and feel comfortable with and prepared to manage these patients in their own practice settings . . . a trial of labor following cesarean section will become widely accepted and practiced only when a significant portion of the obstetric community has had sufficient experience and feels comfortable with this form of management.[28]

It is horrifying that safe, natural alternatives, such as vaginal birth after cesarean, are slow to be accepted, while dubious practices like routine use of electronic fetal monitoring spread like wildfire.

However, repeat cesareans take less time for the physician, particularly if the physician has a policy of remaining with the mother throughout her labor if she has had a previous cesarean. The physician is away from his office more hours. He makes less money with VBAC.

With but few exceptions, obstetricians and hospital staff persons have ignored the many studies disproving the necessity of repeat cesarean. This is extremely perplexing. As Nancy Wainer Cohen and Lois J. Estner state in *Silent Knife*:

> We are frustrated by the multitude of doctors who have obviously done no reading on the subject of VBAC and who confront women with absurd statements such as "It's

too great a risk; I can only guarantee you a healthy baby if you agree to a cesarean..."; "Sure, we'll try it—what difference does a hysterectomy make?"; or "If your uterus ruptures, it means instantaneous death for you and your baby."[29]

It is hard to believe that real physicians could make such statements, which fly in the face of all factual evidence. However, the authors point out that the above are all actual quotes. Such remarks constitute either willful deception on the part of the physician or appalling stupidity.

Dr. D. Sloan polled obstetricians in New York City asking: "Assuming you could be shown documentation and overwhelming evidence of the safety of permitting labor following cesarean section, would you allow this to alter the management of your patients?" Eighty percent responded, "No."[30] This is decidedly strange. It shows, I believe, the utterly unscientific approach of what appears to be a majority of obstetricians (at least in this survey). There is no justifying such an answer. There isn't even a logical explanation.

Nevertheless, one can't blame all repeat cesareans on health professionals. When presented with the option, many mothers have chosen surgical births—many because they fear a failed trial of labor, some because they believe cesarean delivery is easier.[31] Some make their decision because they are afraid of VBAC. This fear stems largely from misconceptions. A few mothers choose elective repeat cesarean for the "convenience" of knowing the date in advance and being assured of having their own physician. This seems an incredible compromise when you consider what is sacrificed for convenience and just how much inconvenience the mother will suffer as a result of major surgery. As Drs. Meier and Porreco point out:

"Neither fear nor convenience constitutes justification for cesarean section."[32] It is the duty, I believe, of childbirth professionals—especially childbirth educators—to acquaint parents with the truth.

With few exceptions, vaginal birth remains the safest, the least traumatic, and the best alternative in every possible way.

Planning a Natural Birth After a Cesarean

The majority of mothers who choose VBAC do birth vaginally. In fact, your chances of birthing naturally after a cesarean are just about as good as those of the woman who has never given birth if: (1) there are no problems in *this* pregnancy, and (2) your cesarean was for a nonrecurrent reason. Most cesareans are done for nonrecurrent reasons, such as the breech position and fetal distress. Recurrent causes include mental illness or severe pelvic contraction (a pelvic opening that is abnormally small). CPD (cephalopelvic disproportion) is not a recurrent reason. This is discussed in more detail ahead.

One study showed an 89 percent VBAC rate among selected patients.[33] In a study conducted by Drs. Meier and Porreco at Kaiser Foundation Hospital in San Diego, out of 207 mothers who had previously had cesareans, 84.5 percent gave birth vaginally.[34] The repeat cesarean rate among these women was therefore 15.5 percent. This is actually *lower* than the national cesarean rate (22.7 percent) for all women. Many other studies have shown similar results.

It is almost always best to opt for vaginal birth rather than elective repeat cesarean. "Everything happened so fast, I lost track of my contractions," recalls Karen about the vaginal birth of her daughter Briana. A sudden incidence of fetal distress almost led to another cesarean. However, within a short time she went from 3 centimeters to full dilation and was pushing. "It was painful. However, although it was pretty rough, I was really glad that I had a VBAC." Even if problems should arise and you end up with a cesarean, the baby will have benefited from labor and have less chance of respiratory distress. And you and your partner will feel you have done all you could for the best possible birth. This will significantly reduce the effects of surgical birth trauma.

To increase your likelihood of a safe, happy, vaginal birth, observe *all* the guidelines in Chapters Four and Five as well as the following:

• Learn about labor (if you haven't experienced it). You should have a realistic idea of labor's pain, and prepare yourself with effective coping methods (effective labor support, mental imagery, and for some mothers, rhythmic breathing patterns).

• Choose a caregiver who will treat you as if you haven't had a cesarean. It is not sufficient if your caregiver is willing to "permit" a trial of labor. Many claim to support VBAC yet treat the laboring mother as if she were planning to give birth while skydiving.

• Perhaps you are mistrustful of a prior caregiver, especially if you believe your cesarean was an unnecessary one. In this case, it is essential to find a more supportive caregiver for this birth.

• If you plan a hospital birth, be sure the hospital you choose supports natural birth after a prior cesarean—and not in name only. Meet the staff and get a feeling for their attitude. The staff of some hospitals recognize that the mother with a prior cesarean has as much likelihood of birthing safely and normally as anyone else. Yet in other hospitals, insensitive staff persons are actually hostile to VBAC mothers. However, as Drs. Meier and Porreco point out, "It is vital for a successful outcome that all care personnel, from physicians to hospital clerks, appear enthusiastic and confident concerning prospects for VBAC."[35]

• Pay special attention to having effective labor support. VBAC mothers need continuous support, even more than women who are laboring for the first time. This is because the VBAC mother tends to be somewhat more anxious. In addition, hospital staff persons tend to be more intervention-prone.

• Consider hiring a professional support person, unless the father is wholly committed to learning about effective support during pregnancy and being actively involved throughout labor.

• Use nonpharmacologic forms of pain relief (mental imagery and effective labor support) in place of pain medication if at all possible (see Chapters Four and Five).

• If you have an electronic fetal monitor, it is best to have intermittent monitoring and be up walking in between.

The VBAC Mother's Special Needs

The overwhelming majority of cesarean mothers planning a vaginal birth are perfectly normal. However, you are in a special situation. Understanding the following facts will help you better plan your birth:

1. The VBAC mother is at greater risk of medical intervention. If healthy, first-time laboring women are sometimes treated like invalids in America, you can imag-

ine how the woman who has had a prior cesarean is often treated (regardless of the fact that she is as healthy as anyone else).

One article describes the *routine* procedures for VBAC at a particular hospital (the article, by the way, is in favor of vaginal birth after a cesarean): The woman is immediately hooked up to EFM on arrival. Intravenous infusion is begun. The mother is restricted from eating or drinking and advised to eat small amounts of ice chips. She is fed an antacid every three to four hours to neutralize stomach acidity (in case of surgery—see the section "The Operation" in Chapter Seven). Supplies are placed right in her room in case of emergency. These include a catheter, urinary drainage bag, and an abdominal prep kit (for preoperative procedures). When membranes rupture, internal electronic fetal monitoring is begun.

With a set-up like this, it is a wonder that any so-called trials of labor succeed!

Mother and baby should, of course, be watched diligently to be sure everything is progressing normally (whether or not the mother has had a previous cesarean). However, this can be done without making her feel as if she were hovering precipitiously on the brink of disaster. You should not have to submit to unnecessary intervention. Nor should you be treated like a high-risk patient because of something that may have happened several years ago. Injudicious medical intervention increases the risk of repeat cesarean.

This underscores the importance of choosing a caregiver and birthing place carefully.

2. The VBAC mother needs confidence and a positive view of birth even more than the woman who hasn't given

birth previously. Many expectant parents lack confidence in the body's ability to birth naturally. Frequently, this is especially true of those who have had prior cesareans.

The language used to describe labor after a previous cesarean—trial of labor—may increase the VBAC mother's anxiety. You may wonder whether or not your so-called trial of labor will be successful.

Many parents fear uterine rupture. Though there is hardly any risk of scar separation, and the risk is the same as it is with elective repeat cesarean, it is nonetheless a real fear.

The mother with a prior cesarean must learn to trust her body. The father, too, should learn as much as he can about birth and develop confidence in his ability to support his partner effectively.

You can develop confidence in several ways. Talk to a caregiver or childbirth educator. Share your feelings with other VBAC and cesarean parents. Consider joining a support group such as C/SEC or the Cesarean Prevention Movement (CPM) (see Resources).

3. The VBAC parent frequently needs to work out unresolved feelings about her prior birth. Many mothers planning a VBAC have strong negative feelings about their cesarean. If these feelings remain unresolved, they can interfere with the present labor and make you and your partner mistrustful of your current caregivers. Therefore, expressing your concerns, anger, frustration, and perhaps grief over your past cesarean is essential.

Many parents find themselves confronting a flood of tears years after the event. Releasing your feelings and forgiving those involved will open the door for healing.

4. The VBAC mother needs an emotionally positive climate in her birthing place. You are much more likely to

labor normally when those around radiate confidence than you are if staff persons, skeptical of VBAC, walk furtively about looking at the clock as if any moment a time bomb might explode.

Unfortunately, many hospitals deprive the VBAC mother the use of a birthing room. Many childbearing centers will not accept VBAC clients. The reason for this is often rooted in state laws or insurance regulations. In any case, this is wholly unfair discrimination. The VBAC mother needs and deserves a comfortable birthing environment just as much as the mother who has never had a cesarean. In fact, she probably needs it more to give her the added emotional reassurance that she is fine and healthy.

Choose the best birthing environment available in your area. If you are not fully comfortable with it, place additional emphasis on creating a positive emotional climate around you with good labor support.

Many mothers are more comfortable having a home VBAC. "For a long time I would cry, thinking I wouldn't be able to have another home birth, though I knew I would be able to birth vaginally," states Phillippa, whose first child was born at home, her second child by cesarean. "I couldn't imagine having the same wonderful experience in the hospital that I had had at home. I realize some say that their hospital experience was fine. But with my situation, if I had to go back to the hospital, I'm sure it would reactivate the bad memories of my cesarean and interfere with my labor." Fortunately, after doing much research, Phillippa discovered that she could have a safe home birth and was able to find a midwife to assist her.

If you cannot find a caregiver to attend a home VBAC, consult the NAPSAC *Directory of Alternate Birth Services Consumer Guide* (see Resources).

Common Medical Guidelines for Managing a VBAC Labor

If you are healthy, you should be treated as though you never had a cesarean. However, you are lucky if you find a caregiver who approaches VBAC this way.

No hard-and-fast rules are applicable for every mother expecting a baby after a previous surgical delivery. Guidelines vary with the mother's situation and the policies of her caregiver and hospital. Some of the commonly observed guidelines do not make much sense. Many are far too restrictive and rule out a great many perfectly healthy "candidates" for vaginal birth. You may encounter any or all of the following:

- *The mother is informed of the risks and informed consent obtained.* She should always be informed of risks—including those associated with electronic fetal monitoring, Pitocin, repeat cesarean, and so forth. However, stressing the need to inform the mother of the risks of VBAC seems rather curious since they are far less than those of repeat cesarean.
- *The previous cesarean was done for a nonrecurrent reason* (such as breech presentation) rather than a recurrent cause (such as absolute pelvic contraction).
- *The mother is admitted to a hospital as early as possible in labor.* Though this is a common policy, the VBAC mother with a low transverse uterine incision shouldn't have to be admitted to the hospital any earlier than the mother who hasn't had a prior cesarean, unless there are complications in *this* pregnancy. In fact, this practice actually has disadvantages. As Drs. Porreco and Meier point out, being under intensive surveillance "can needlessly alarm attendants and lead to harmful interven-

tion that may result in a repeat CS [cesarean section]."[36] The mother with a classic uterine incision, however, should be admitted to the hospital as soon as labor begins. In her case, intravenous feeding may also be justified.

• *Facilities and nursing and surgical personnel should be available to perform an immediate cesarean if the need arises.* However, facilities required for VBAC emergencies are really no different from those required for any other obstetrical emergency. According to Dr. Luella Klein, former president of the American College of Obstetricians and Gynecologists: "Trial of labor requires the same services that keep other laboring patients and their infants safe. Emergencies arising from hemorrhage, prolapsed cord, or fetal distress will occur wherever babies are delivered and will occur more frequently than symptomatic rupture of uterus does in patients properly selected for trial of labor."[37] Meanwhile, if the VBAC mother opts for home birth, she should make the same back-up plans regarding a hospital as she would had she never had a cesarean.

• *The duration of labor should conform to averages.* However, the mother planning a vaginal birth after cesarean is just as likely to have a longer or shorter than average labor as anyone else. One can't very well expect her to conform to "averages" just because she has a uterine scar. If the mother is healthy, and there are no signs of fetal distress, there is no reason to put a time limit on her labor.

• *The mother must labor without medication.* This is so that she can feel warning pain prior to uterine rupture. However, numerous studies have shown that abdominal pain is not a reliable sign of uterine rupture.[38] Therefore, the mother should have the final choice about whether or not to use medication. Telling a mother she can't have pain-relief medication is tantamount to exerting unfair pressure on her to choose a repeat cesarean. As Drs. Porreco and Meier point out, "Suggesting without good reason to VBAC patients that they will be unable to take advantage of a particular analgesic technique during labor unjustifiably makes repeat CS [cesarean section] more attractive."[39]

On the other hand, it is always better for the course of labor and the health of the baby to try nonpharmacological pain relief before resorting to medication.

• *The physician should be present throughout the mother's labor.* This medical guideline is one reason physicians are reluctant to get involved with VBACs. According to the Canadian Consensus Report, the continuous presence of the physician is not necessary during VBAC labors any more than it is during other labor.[40] In fact, according to Dr. Don Creevy, a prominent West Coast obstetrician with a natural approach to childbirth, "The continual presence of a physician is probably a disadvantage, because he or she might make the mother nervous."

• *The mother cannot use Pitocin for inducing or augmenting labor.* This is because Pitocin supposedly increases the possibility of uterine rupture. However, according to Drs. Janet M. Horenstein and Jeffrey P. Phelan of Women's Hospital, Los Angeles County/University of Southern California Medical Center: "Use of oxytocin with VBAC mothers is a safe and reasonable consideration."[41]

As mentioned in Chapter Five, Pitocin should remain a last resort only after all other methods of inducing or augmenting labor have first been tried.

• *The mother should have EFM.* As discussed in Chapter Three, EFM is one of the contributing causes of unnecessary surgery. Though the mother should be monitored carefully, this doesn't mean it has to be done electronically.

• *Forceps are used to shorten second stage.* A few obstetricians adhere to this policy because they believe it helps prevent uterine rupture. However, others reserve the use of forceps only for such indications as would warrant instrumental delivery if the mother has had no prior cesarean.

Fortunately, these and other requirements are beginning to relax. The policies of physicians and hospitals are changing as more and more health professionals discover for themselves that VBAC is indeed the best alternative. Meanwhile, if you don't fit within the medical guidelines of those practicing in your area, you may have to work harder to find a suitable caregiver and birthing place. Some couples even have to relocate temporarily or travel a long distance. One issue of the Cesarean Prevention Movement's *Clarion* included a moving story of a couple who traveled from Alaska to California to receive the kind of care they wanted. However, the effort the parents spend planning a vaginal birth is rarely regretted.

IF YOUR PREVIOUS CESAREAN WAS FOR CPD

A previous cesarean for CPD (cephalopelvic disproportion—see Chapter Two) is never a contraindication for vaginal delivery during a subsequent pregnancy.

As stated previously, it is nearly impossible to determine true CPD, since the mother's pelvic bones and the baby's head mold to one another during birth. Moreover, CPD is usually not caused exclusively by the baby's size or the size of the maternal pelvis, but is often a relationship of the three Ps—passenger, passage, and powers. For example, CPD may be a combination of poor fetal position and inefficient contractions.

Your chance of delivering vaginally is slightly reduced if you have had a cesarean for CPD. However, it is still excellent. Numerous studies have proven that the overwhelming majority of mothers previously sectioned for CPD may still birth normally.[42] In an exhaustive study by Drs. Meier and Porreco, 78 percent of mothers who initially had cesareans as a result of failure to progress in labor for CPD subsequently gave birth vaginally.[43] In another study by Dr. Richard Paul and his associates at the Los Angeles County/University of Southern California Medical Center at Women's Hospital, 77 percent of mothers who previously had cesareans for CPD gave birth vaginally.[44] The rate of uterine dehiscence (scar separation) in this study was no higher among VBAC mothers than in those who had planned cesareans.

Often, the babies who are born vaginally are just as large or *larger* than those for which the mother previously had a cesarean.

If You Have Had More than One Cesarean

Whether you've had one prior cesarean or many, your chances of birthing vaginally are excellent. There is not a great deal of evidence available regarding vaginal birth after multiple cesareans. However, the limited research that has been done is quite encouraging.

According to Drs. Porreco and Meier, available evidence now suggests that a trial of labor following previous multiple cesareans is "both reasonable and safe."[45] Of the mothers with multiple cesareans these two physicians have studied, 81 percent delivered vaginally. Pitocin was used as medically indicated, and epidural anesthesia was available to those who chose it. One might expect an even higher rate of success if anesthesia was avoided and if natural means of labor augmentation, rather than Pitocin, were used.

The mother who has had more than one prior cesarean may have a somewhat lower chance of birthing vaginally than the mother with only one previous cesarean. In one study conducted by Drs. Riva and Teich,[46] mothers who had multiple cesareans had a 66 percent VBAC success rate, compared to an 80 percent rate among mothers with one prior surgical birth. Curiously, in another study conducted by Dr. Luis Saldana and his associates, the VBAC success rate was actually higher among mothers who had multiple cesareans (58 percent compared to 34 percent).[47] However, both these studies included only a small number of mothers, and one cannot draw definitive conclusions from either.

Meanwhile, there is no evidence of increased maternal or perinatal risk from trial of labor after previous multiple cesareans.[48]

OTHER SITUATIONS

Many physicians have suggested that various factors increase the risk of VBAC. These include: placental location, fever after the prior cesarean, a large baby, twins, breech presentation, time lapse since the prior cesarean, and multiple cesarean births. There is no evidence that any of these factors increases the risk of uterine rupture.

AFTER THE BABY IS BORN

The postpartum period after a natural birth is similar whether a mother has had a previous cesarean or not.

Many caregivers, however, do an internal exam to palpate the uterine scar to see if there has been a dehiscence with neither symptoms nor hemorrhage. Yet more often than not, such defects, when they are discovered, are not treated in any way. Therefore, the benefit of the exam, as one study put it, "is obscure."[49] For the patient, the exam is both uncomfortable (though it only lasts a minute or so) and unnecessary. Its only value seems to be theoretical—that is, to determine whether or not there has been a dehiscence. Dr. Creevy states that he gave up the practice of examining VBAC mothers as "unnecessary at best." If you wish to avoid the exam, discuss this with your caregiver.

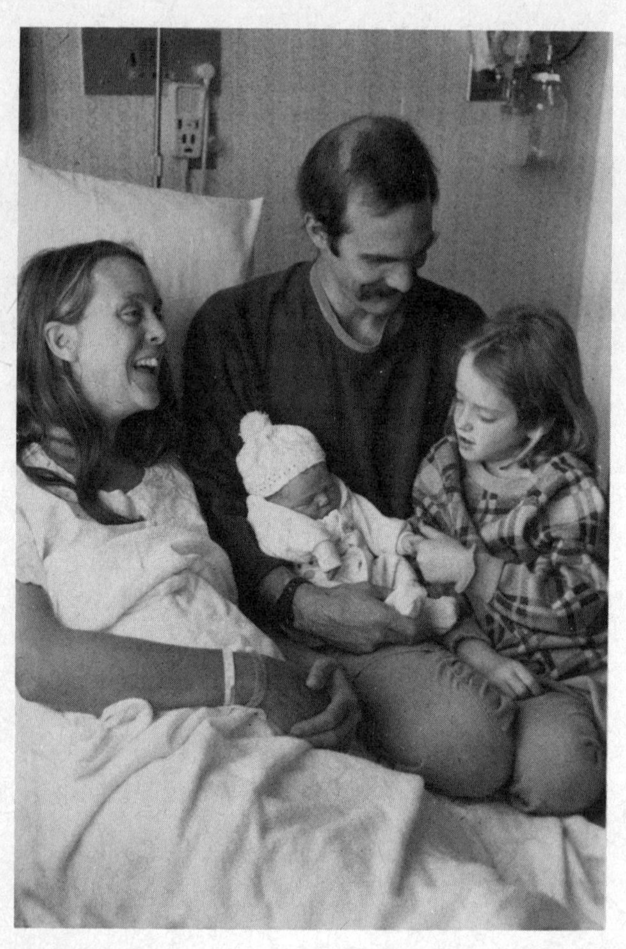

chapter seven

If a Cesarean Is Necessary

Though every attempt should be made to avoid surgical birth, a cesarean section is occasionally necessary to preserve the health of mother and/or baby. The reasons for a necessary cesarean are discussed in Chapter Two. Though one can't minimize the reality of surgery or the loss of a vaginal birth, a necessary cesarean need not be an entirely negative experience.

Whether surgery is planned in advance or the decision is made at the last minute during labor, you can take simple commonsense steps to make your birth a joyful event and your postcesarean recovery as smooth as possible.

Should a cesarean prove necessary, observing the steps in Chapters Three and Four will not have been wasted. They will reduce surgical birth trauma for the entire family. Besides, you will have done all you could to avoid *unnecessary* surgical birth. This alone can greatly minimize emotional trauma. In addition, having explored all your options and planned your birth wisely, including carefully choosing a caregiver and birthing place, your likelihood of the best possible cesarean recovery will be greater.

Additional ways to reduce surgical birth trauma include: making informed decisions; remaining with your partner throughout the experience; being as active a participant as possible under the circumstances; prolonged parent-infant contact directly following delivery; breastfeeding immediately or as soon after birth as possible; and arranging for the help of family and/or friends during the postpartum recovery era.

ESSENTIAL CHOICES

Cesarean parents are frequently unaware that they have several choices that influence their birth experience and postpartum recovery. Rarely is there a life-threatening situation when medical experts must make decisions so rapidly that there is no time for the mother and father to have input.

The most important choices regard:

- The time of birth, that is, whether you have a scheduled cesarean or wait until labor begins.
- The type of anesthesia to be used.
- How the father will be involved during surgery and immediately afterward.
- Parent-infant contact after birth.

Making informed decisions about these issues and choosing the best alternatives will help reduce surgical birth trauma.

THE SCHEDULED CESAREAN

Most cesareans are unplanned. The decision to perform surgery is made in labor. Only if it is planned in advance do you have a choice about timing. However, surgical birth should be planned only after you have explored all your options and are firmly convinced that vaginal birth is truly inadvisable.

Unless there is a strong reason for immediate delivery (such as severe maternal illness or a complication such as a prolapsed cord), it is best to wait until labor begins naturally. This way, you are sure the baby is mature and the lungs will function properly at birth. Numerous studies have conclusively shown that the risk of breathing difficulties and related lung disease is far less if the mother waits until labor begins.[1] This is so even when the baby is mature. Full-term babies delivered without the benefits of labor also risk lung problems. A group of physicians at the Indiana School of Medicine in Indianapolis point out: "Much of the respiratory distress associated with elective cesarean section, especially repeat cesarean section, might be prevented if the mother were allowed to begin labor spontaneously before the cesarean section was performed."[2]

The chance of infection with repeat cesarean is somewhat higher if the mother undergoes labor first. However, it is no greater than the risk of infection among mothers having a primary (first-time) cesarean.[3]

TYPES OF ANESTHESIA

Two basic types of anesthesia are used for cesarean surgery: *general anesthesia*, in which the mother is unconscious, and *regional anesthesia*, in which the mother is anesthetized but able to be conscious for the birth. In addition, acupuncture is occasionally used.

General Anesthesia

General anesthesia is occasionally used in emergencies when speed is essential to save the life of mother or baby as, for example, in the event of a severe case of placenta previa involving massive maternal bleeding. Some low-back problems, certain allergies, and hypotension may also contraindicate the use of regional anesthesia. However, some women prefer and choose general over regional anesthesia because they would rather not be awake during their operation.

When it is time to administer the anesthesic, pentothal sodium is added to the IV. It then takes only fifteen to twenty seconds to become unconscious: Once the mother is asleep, endotracheal intubation, in which a tube is passed down the throat and into the windpipe to prevent aspiration of stomach contents, is begun. (This sometimes causes a mild sore throat for a few days.) Nitrous oxide and oxygen are then given to maintain the anesthesia. The mother wakes up when the surgery is completed.

The major disadvantage is the very slight risk of aspirating stomach contents, possibly leading to severe pneumonia and, very rarely, maternal death. Other disadvantages are that the mother is not awake for the birth and that often mother and baby are too groggy to participate in the bonding process for several hours afterward.

In most hospitals, the father is not permitted in the delivery room when general anesthesia is used. However, some hospitals and physicians will make an exception. The father should be allowed to be present at the birth regardless of the type of anesthesia used and whether the mother is unconscious or awake.

Regional Anesthesia

This includes both *spinal* and *epidural* anesthesia. Both numb the body from the chest to the toes and render the area temporarily immobile.

Most cesarean mothers prefer regional anesthesia so

they can be awake to experience the birth and see the baby immediately afterward. Several studies have shown that mothers who have regional anesthesia tend to have a more positive perception of their cesarean experience than those who have had general. This does not imply, however, that you can't have a fulfilling postpartum experience if you have had general anesthesia.

With regional anesthesia, you may feel pressure, tugging, and pulling sensations during surgery, but there should be no pain. If you do feel pain, simply tell the physician so the anesthesia can be adjusted.

For both spinal and epidural, the mother lies on her side with her back curled toward the anesthesiologist. The spinal, involves only a single injection. Spinals are sometimes followed by *spinal headaches* requiring the mother to lie flat on her bed for eight hours or so. This may be the result of the leakage of a small quantity of cerebrospinal fluid through the puncture holes. However, spinal headaches are less common today as a result of the use of small-gauge needles to administer the anesthesic.

Most consider epidural the anesthesia of choice for a cesarean because there is less chance of aftereffects and it is easier to control. A very thin hollow tube is inserted into the back and taped in place for the duration of the surgery so that more anesthesic can be injected as needed. Occasionally, there is a "window," that is, an area not fully anesthetized. However, this is rare, and if it does occur, the anesthesiologist will simply adjust the anesthetic.

Local anesthesia, consisting of several injections in the abdomen, can be effective but is rarely used in this country.

THE OPERATION

A cesarean section generally takes about an hour from start to finish. However, the baby is usually born within the first fifteen minutes. The remaining time is spent stitching the incisions.

Although you and your partner are bound to feel anything but relaxed, there is usually plenty of time to ask questions and make informed decisions. However, in extreme emergencies (such as severe abruptio placantae or prolapsed cord), the procedure is speeded up.

Preoperative Procedures

The following procedures are done shortly before surgery, usually in the labor room. However, in some hospitals they may be done after you have been moved to the operating room (this is usually the delivery room).

The abdomen is shaved. An IV is started, and a catheter is inserted through the urethra into the bladder to remove fluid from the bladder. Antacid is given to neutralize stomach acids.

In many hospitals, mothers are routinely given sedation. This causes grogginess during and after the birth for both mother and baby. If you prefer to be fully alert, request no preoperative medication.

When you are moved to the delivery room and onto the delivery table, routine procedures generally include strapping the arms to two boards extended on either side of the table (like the wings of an airplane) or to your sides. This prevents inadvertently touching the sterile area. You can request that one arm be left free (or loosely strapped) or that the strap be removed immediately after birth so you can touch your baby.

Sometimes, the leads to a cardiac monitor are placed on your chest to give continual heartbeat feedback during the operation. A blood-pressure cuff is attached to your arm so your pressure can be checked frequently.

The anesthesic will then be administered and surgery begun.

The father may be allowed to be present during preoperative procedures. This is certainly an anxious time, and the mother will benefit from her partner's continual presence and support. Usually, however, the father is asked to remain in the waiting room until the mother is fully prepared and surgery ready to begin (about one-half hour or so). If being together without separation is important to you, be sure the hospital you choose permits this. You can discuss this point with your caregiver.

The Birth

Shortly after surgery is begun, you will see your baby. Ask your physician to show you the baby as soon as she is born. Unless there is a grave emergency, this should be routine. The baby will then be examined by a nurse or pediatrician. You can request that the exam be done near you so you can observe it. The baby's nose and throat may have to be suctioned, as babies born surgically often need to have mucus suctioned from the air passageways.

After the exam, the father should take the baby and hold her close to you. You can caress the infant with your hands (if they are free) or with your face, kiss her, smell the fresh odor of the newborn, and enjoy eye-to-eye contact.

The baby will keep her eyes closed in a brightly lit delivery room. She has been used to the near-dark womb, and bright light hurts the sensitive newborn's eyes. However, bright lights are necessary during cesarean surgery. Cupping a hand just above the baby's eyes sometimes encourages the infant to open them.

If there is need for immediate pediatric care, the baby is taken to an intensive care unit (ICU). Depending on the parents' preference, the father can either remain with the mother while she is being stitched or accompany the child to the ICU. If he goes to the ICU, he can later share the baby's first actions with the mother. After the mother is stitched, she can also go to the ICU on a rolling bed to see the baby.

The Father's Role During Surgical Birth

"It meant everything to me to have David there," said one mother recalling the cesarean birth of her son. "We were mostly quiet, but he was right there with me. It was calming and soothing and we were looking at each other. The baby screamed as soon as he came out. I was able to hear that scream and it was wonderful."[4]

To most mothers, the father's presence during a cesarean makes a world of difference. Several studies have demonstrated that his being there has a positive effect on the birth experience.[5] Pediatrician T. Berry Brazelton stresses that the family has a better chance of raising the baby in a nurturing way if the couple shares the birth.[6] In addition, being present affects the father's own experience and may help him better adapt to his new family.

During cesarean surgery, the father has an especially important role. His very presence can lessen the mother's fear. Sharing the experience keeps both parents focused on the birth rather than the surgical procedure.

The father does not have to observe the surgery. He sits next to his partner's head, and a screen placed between the mother's head and abdomen blocks both parents' view. Of course, if he wishes to observe, he can simply stand up.

Sometimes, a father takes photos of the delivery. If he plans to do this, he should let the caregiver know and be sure not to get so caught up in taking pictures that he forgets to support his partner.

Needless to say, the father will not be as active as he could be during a vaginal birth. He will miss the thrill of touching the baby as it is being born, of perhaps "catching" the baby himself, and of cutting the umbilical cord. However, his presence is still essential.

The most effective support he can give is just being by his partner's side, perhaps holding her hand (if it is not strapped) and sharing the tense moments before the child is born. George, one new father, said, "I felt that my role was reassuring Diane, holding her hand, keeping her calm, just talking to her." One mother recalls: "He held my hand during the surgery and told me I was not alone. He spoke for me when I could not talk and when the baby came out he held her for me."[7]

As mentioned before, unless there is a problem requiring immediate pediatric intervention, the father should take the baby in his arms as soon as possible after birth. He and his partner can then begin taking part immediately in the parent-infant attachment process.

Since the majority of cesareans are unplanned, you should always find out about hospital policies regarding the father's presence during cesarean sections before making a final decision about your birthing place. Most hospitals today welcome parental participation. However, a few still do not permit fathers in the delivery room during surgery. Avoid such institutions. Every father has a right to witness the birth of his child, whether that child is born vaginally or surgically. I strongly urge all parents not to support any hospital that refuses to honor this right.

Frequently, the anesthesiology department's policy prohibits fathers from attending cesareans. The obstetrician may be willing, but the anesthesiologist not. Some feel that fathers will react poorly or get in the way. However, this is not true. Meanwhile, any policy that prohibits fathers from attending preparatory procedures or the birth, or that restricts visiting time afterward, is inappropriate. No health professional, regardless of his or her motive, should separate family members before, during, or after birth.

Parent-Infant Contact After Birth

Early and prolonged contact between parent and infant is important whether the baby is born normally or surgically.

The first hour or so following birth is a sensitive time for mothers and babies. After an unmedicated birth, the baby is usually quite alert. Both mother and baby are especially receptive to one another. Prolonged contact promotes the parent-infant attachment process (bonding), helps the mother adjust to motherhood, and reduces the likelihood of postpartum depression. It enables the mother to take on her caretaking role more smoothly. Studies have shown that it is also associated with a woman's self-confidence in her ability to mother and the later healthy development of the child. In addition, studies have shown that breastfeeding success is correlated with early maternal-infant contact.

According to one postcesarean study, mothers who have early contact with their infants seem to exhibit significantly more maternal behavior in caretaking during the first or second postpartum day, as well as when the infant is one month old, than do mothers who have only brief contact.[8] Yet odd as it may seem, some hospitals routinely separate mothers and infants following vaginal as well as cesarean birth. Without doubt, this is one of the most bizarre and inhuman childbearing customs of all times.

Cesarean-born babies are frequently placed in an intensive-care nursery for twenty-four hours after birth. Having lost the benefits of a natural birth, they often do have more trouble breathing. However, unless there is a serious medical problem, separating mother and baby is wholly unnecessary. Fortunately, this practice is falling by the wayside.

Arrange to be with your infant immediately after birth unless there are complications requiring immediate pediatric intervention. Obviously, your freedom to relate to your baby will be restricted after surgery. However, you still can and should establish parent-infant contact. The father can help you while bonding with the child himself.

By the same token, you should not be forced to care for your child before you are ready. You may first have to meet your own needs. Though this seems to contradict the previous statements about the importance of early maternal-infant contact, it is frequently more important for the mother to come to terms with her surgical birth before taking care of her baby. Let your emotions and physical needs be your guide. You will feel able to mother your baby soon.

Needless to say, bonding is not a once-and-forever thing. Developing parent-infant attachment is an ongoing process. Cesarean parents are sometimes separated from their infants as a result of medical problems needing immediate attention, the use of general anesthesia, or just the need to be by themselves for a while. If this occurs, simply make up for lost time as soon as you are able.

The Recovery Room

When surgery is complete, you are taken to a recovery room (in some hospitals directly to the postpartum unit), where you remain two or three hours until the anesthesia wears off and your condition is stabilized. The father should accompany the mother to the recovery room and remain with her and the baby—save for time out for the exciting phone calls. During these first few hours, you and your partner can begin to share your feelings, disappointments, and joys.

In the recovery room, a nurse checks temperature, pulse, blood pressure, respiration, incision site, and vaginal discharge. Even if you have birthed abdominally, *lochia* (postbirth discharge) will flow and should be checked. You will probably also be offered a bed bath, a toothbrush, and mouthwash to freshen up.

If you have had general anesthesia, you will feel groggy for a while. If you have had an epidural or spinal, a nurse will ask you to wiggle your toes, move your feet, and bend your knees. Your legs may begin to tingle as regional anesthesia wears off. Following spinal anesthesia, you may have to remain flat on your back for eight to twelve hours to prevent postspinal headache.

You may experience discomfort ranging from mild to severe at the incision site. If you have pain, don't hesitate to ask for pain medication. The amount that gets to the baby during breastfeeding is negligible and won't have any long-lasting effects. However, it is important that you are not uncomfortable and are able to enjoy the baby without unnecessary pain.

If you have had tranquilizers with the anesthesia, you may need to sleep for a while. Sheila, one new mother, said, "Shortly after delivery with an epidural, I fell into a deep sleep in the recovery room while my husband Dave sat nearby holding the baby. It gave me a peaceful feeling watching him get to know our new daughter, Amy, as I drifted off to sleep."

Spend as much time as possible with your baby in the recovery room. This will minimize the effects of surgical birth trauma on you, your baby, and your relationship.

Ask that your baby be unwrapped and placed on your abdomen so you can have skin-to-skin contact. Your partner can do this for you.

Begin breastfeeding—the earlier the better. Your partner can help you get into a comfortable position and hold the baby as needed. Of course, a nurse is also available to do this. However, it is better if the father is involved during this early stage.

If you find yourself very tired and want to rest, your partner can hold the baby close to you, or the baby can be placed in an infant warmer next to your bed.

YOUR POSTPARTUM STAY

After two or three hours in the recovery room, you will be taken to the postpartum unit. Here your hospital stay may range from three to seven days. Some parents prefer early discharge (within three days) and feel more comfortable at home. If this is your preference, discuss it with your physician. Other mothers are overwhelmed and prefer to remain in the hospital.

For the first twenty-four to forty-eight hours, your IV and catheter may remain in place. The IV is needed to supply fluids until your condition is stable. (The amount of time this takes varies from mother to mother.) The catheter is needed to drain the bladder, which remains sluggish for a while after surgery and anesthesia. Your diet will consist first of liquids, then gradually change to regular meals.

A nurse will check vital signs (temperature, pulse, blood

pressure, and respiration), the dressing, your uterus, and vaginal discharge.

The nurse will ask you either to cough or "huff" to clear the lungs of excess mucus that accumulates after surgery and to help prevent pneumonia. Huffing is more comfortable and is as effective as coughing. Simply take in a deep breath and exhale with an audible "huff." As you do so, you can press a towel or pillow firmly against your incision to ease discomfort.

Shift your position in bed often until you are up and walking. This facilitates blood circulation, promotes healing, and decreases the likelihood of gas pains.

You should also do *abdominal tightening* to strengthen the abdominal muscles, promote healing, and help prevent gas pains:

> Inhale deeply so that the belly rises on the in-breath.
>
> Exhale evenly and steadily, tightening the abdominal muscles as you do so.
>
> Repeat 4–5 times every hour.

Don't worry about the incision. It will not pull apart.

Your partner can remind you to shift in bed and do abdominal tightening.

After surgical birth, simple activities will probably be uncomfortable for a while. However, medication is always available. If the pain is severe, consult your physician.

Getting Out of Bed

You should get out of bed and walk around within the first twenty-four hours after birth unless your physician advises otherwise. Getting up early minimizes the chance of developing a blood clot and promotes healing.

Don't try to stand up alone the first time. A nurse or your partner should assist you. Afterward, your partner can be there for you to lean on when you walk.

Once you are up, try to stand straight and tall even though this may be uncomfortable at first. This promotes healing. Cesarean mothers frequently adopt a stooped-over posture while walking (referred to as the "cesarean shuffle") to protect the incision. But the stitches will not pull apart.

Rooming-In

You, your baby, and your partner have had a rocky birth. To lessen further trauma, it is essential to make the postpartum period as normal as possible under the circumstances.

Rooming-in—that is, mother and baby remain in the same room throughout their hospital stay—facilitates breastfeeding, aids in the development of the maternal-infant relationship, and lessens the likelihood of postpartum depression. Besides, a newborn belongs with her mother. The central nursery, in which babies are placed in sterile bassinets under bright lights like exotic plants, is hardly an appropriate place to begin extrauterine life.

Underscoring the importance of rooming-in doesn't mean the parents must feel obligated to be with their child all of the time. In fact, as the weeks pass the parents will probably want to spend time alone together away from the baby. However, being together the first few sensitive days is important.

Rooming-in needn't be an all-or-nothing affair. If you want time by yourself and don't feel up to caring for the baby, you can always ask a nurse to remove her every now and then.

Since the cesarean mother is often uncomfortable and not as mobile as the mother who births vaginally, the father can take on the greater share of baby care—diapering, bathing, holding the baby, and so forth. Nurses, of course, are available to do this, but it is better for the parents to learn to take care of their baby as soon as possible. Homecoming will then be much less traumatic, and both parents will feel more confident.

Breastfeeding

The American Academy of Pediatrics recommends that breast milk be the infant's primary food source for the first six months of life. It is the ideal and only perfectly designed food for human babies.

Cesarean babies need the physical and emotional benefits of breastfeeding just as much as do babies born vaginally. Nursing should therefore be established as soon as possible, even if it is a little difficult at first. Nursing may have to be delayed, of course, if the baby is distressed and in need of immediate care or if the mother is too tired. Though it is preferable to begin nursing shortly after birth, it is never too late.

If you haven't made up your mind whether to breast- or bottle-feed, it is best to begin nursing. You can always change your mind later and switch to the bottle. However, it is more difficult (but by no means impossible) to switch to the breast once bottle feedings have begun.

To avoid discomfort, hold the baby in a position that avoids direct pressure on the incision. Two comfortable positions are:

Side-lying. Lie on one side with the baby cradled in your arms and facing you. Use pillows to support your back, belly, and perhaps your upper leg. When you finish nursing from one side, roll over and nurse from the other breast.

Your partner or a nurse can hold the baby while you shift position.

To burp the baby, roll over on your back and hold the baby up.

Sitting. Place a pillow over the stitches before cradling the baby in your arm. Sit with bent knees to lessen strain on the abdomen. The hospital bed can be adjusted to a comfortable position.

Relieving the Common Postcesarean Discomforts

Discomfort from the incision, as already mentioned, can be relieved with medication. Be sure your physician is aware that you are nursing so he can prescribe a pain medication that will have minimal effects on the baby. The discomfort will be much less within a week.

Gas Pain

For most cesarean mothers, this is the major discomfort, ranging from mild to severe. As a result of both anesthesia and the surgical procedure, bowel function is delayed for a while. Excess gas may build up as the intestines start to work by the second or third postpartum day. The gas build-up is actually a positive sign that things are getting back to normal.

To relieve

Rock in a rocking chair while nursing your baby. Intervals of rocking help many cesarean mothers prevent or reduce gas pains.

Avoid carbonated beverages, apple juice (which can be gas-producing), iced drinks (however, ice chips are fine), and drinking through a straw (which can increase air intake). Avoid any other foods that normally cause you to form gas.

Move about in bed often. Roll from side to side.

Walk frequently.

Do abdominal tightening (see page 166).

Lie on your left side, draw up your knees, and massage your abdomen from right to left.

If the discomfort is severe and none of these methods relieve it, tell your caregiver or a nurse. Sometimes a thin tube can be placed up the rectum to relieve the gas. This is not painful.

Shoulder Pain

Many mothers experience pain in one or both shoulders. This is caused by blood and/or air collecting under the diaphragm. The pain is deferred through nerve passages to the shoulder. This passes in two or three days.

Medication is the most effective relief.

INVOLVING SIBLINGS

Other children should have a chance to see you and the baby shortly after birth (not a day or two later). They, too, must make major emotional adjustments when a new baby comes. They, too, have a right to be included in this life-transforming event.

Siblings should be allowed to greet the baby face to face and hold the baby, not merely view the infant through the glass window of a nursery (unless, of course, there is a genuine complication requiring the infant to be in intensive care).

Being separated from his parents during this very sensitive time is a traumatic experience for a child. Yet in spite of this, some hospitals actually restrict sibling visits—

forbidding the child to see his own mother or hold his own baby brother or sister. Strange as it may seem, some of the very hospitals that do so claim to be "family-centered"—a testimony to the often empty meaning of hospital advertising. Avoid any institution that does not welcome children without restriction. I recommend that parents do this whether or not they have other children. Institutions with such policies should not be patronized.

MEETING THE SPECIAL NEEDS OF THE CESAREAN MOTHER

The cesarean mother is in a unique position. She must recover both from having given birth and from major abdominal surgery. She must begin taking care of another while she is in need of care herself. She has all the needs and conflicting emotions of the mother who has given birth vaginally. And she has the needs of the postoperative patient.

As a result, cesarean mothers are often not immediately enthusiastic about taking care of the baby. They must think of meeting their own needs. The father's presence during labor, the operation, recovery, and during the postpartum hospital stay will help immensely. Reviewing events and discussing feelings is also important to help the mother deal with her experience. Early maternal-infant contact can facilitate the bond between parent and child. The family-centered birthing atmosphere is essential for a positive postcesarean experience.

The new cesarean mother needs extra help both in the hospital and at home. Of course, in the hospital nurses are available to give expert care around the clock. But professionals, however sensitive, can't substitute for familiar faces. Birth is a family affair, and what the mother needs is her own family—above all, her partner.

By the same token, too many visitors can exhaust the new cesarean mother. The father can help limit their number.

After any birth, the new mother usually feels vulnerable and dependent. These feelings are magnified for the cesarean mother. She needs her partner more than ever. The father's simple actions can be a tremendous benefit.

The most important thing is remaining together as much as possible. In some hospitals, the new family can stay together around the clock, and the father rooms-in with the mother and baby—which is the way it should be. This, unfortunately, is not yet available in most hospitals. However, the father should visit as often as possible.

Besides taking the greater share of baby care, the father can bring the baby to the mother, help her change position as comfortable, rub her back, and brush her hair if she wishes.

The father should take at least a week's paternity leave to be with his partner both in the hospital and at home. Financial concerns loom large after a baby is born (especially via cesarean), and the father may not be paid for the time he takes. However, at this time his emotional support takes priority. He should be with his unfolding family. No work is more important than this.

At home, the father shouldn't allow himself to become so busy with housekeeping and cooking that he forgets to spend time with his family. Though his help is needed, his presence is the most important thing.

Arrange for help at home, and don't refuse any offers. Family members and friends can assist tremendously by helping out with housekeeping, thus freeing some of the father's time.

If you have no family or close friend living nearby, you might consider hiring a postpartum aid. In addition to doing light housekeeping and preparing meals, these persons specialize in the sensitive postpartum period and can assist with breastfeeding and parenting concerns. As more and more parents opt for early discharge, the services of these unique professions is becoming increasingly common. Ask your childbirth educator for a reference.

Regardless of how many others are helping, the father should still remain at home. No one can substitute for him.

Bear in mind that the father, too, has special needs. He, too, has crossed the one-way bridge to parenthood. Though it is the mother who has undergone major surgery, the father too is probably profoundly affected by cesarean birth. Sharing their feelings will help both parents adjust.

POSTCESAREAN EMOTIONS

As stated earlier, parents react to cesarean surgery in different ways. Some don't seem to mind the fact of surgery. "I didn't feel bad about the birth at any point," recalls Karen. "I was glad I was awake, although I felt I was missing something." Others are quite disappointed that they missed a vaginal birth.

Knowing that you've done everything you could to avoid an *unnecessary* cesarean helps. "Things didn't turn out the way Ray and I planned," said Pamela after her cesarean. "But we both did the best we could. For that I am truly satisfied."

The joy, the awe, and the elation that follow vaginal birth often follow a cesarean as well. "It was wonderful greeting our child the instant she was born," said Julie, who had a cesarean as a result of placenta previa. "At that moment it didn't matter how she was born." Her husband, Ken, agreed. "I was so happy to see our daughter Cheryl safe and healthy. It was an unforgettable experience."

However, after the initial wave of elation that so often crowns the birth of a child, both parents may suffer grief at the loss of a normal birth. Margie, whose daughter was born via cesarean after a diagnosis of CPD, writes: "Often . . . especially at night, my mind would wander off and try to piece together the birth, hospital stay, and my feelings about it all. I felt disappointment, confusion, betrayal, anger, and an awful lot of self-pity."[9]

For those who have hoped, planned, and prepared for a normal birth, a cesarean can be emotionally devastating. Recalling his wife's cesarean while he was in the waiting room, Kenneth acknowledges: "I felt utter and profound dejection, disillusionment, and despair . . . The next four days were virtually a living hell for me, as I struggled to come to grips with, to integrate, our trauma."[10]

Joe, another father, states: "The whole experience was a nightmare. We were planning on having a home birth for the second child. When we were told we were going to have a cesarean, we were both devastated." Joe and Phillippa's third child was born vaginally.

Both parents frequently have more difficulty "taking in" their child—one reason rooming-in is so important. Even if the cesarean is necessary and comes as a relief after long hours of hard labor, there is still disappointment. There are conflicting feelings—of gratitude that the baby is safe, of depression, anger, bitterness, and perhaps self-blame. "Sure I was happy the baby was O.K.," recalls Pamela after her son was born surgically as a result of fetal distress. "But I was also miserable."

Cesarean mothers often feel that they have failed. Reassurance is important. A woman has not failed as a result of a cesarean. She has become a mother.

Many parents remain upset for weeks, even months afterward. Releasing the emotional pain and perhaps anger is essential for complete recovery. It is sometimes helpful for the mother and her partner to discuss the details and recall the events that led up to the cesarean decision. This is especially so if the mother had general anesthesia and has only a foggy memory of the events before and after surgery.

Sharing your feelings with understanding friends can help. Childbirth professionals are also sometimes helpful. An increasing number are aware that there is more to having a baby than coming through the experience alive. However, not all are equally supportive or understanding. Many are not aware of the unique and powerful feelings of cesarean parents.

Don't hesitate to contact a support group such as C/SEC, which provides emotional support for cesarean families (see Resources).

Meanwhile, forgiveness is a powerful form of self-healing. This means forgiving the obstetrician, the nurses, perhaps your own partner if he didn't provide what you consider adequate support, forgiving anyone involved. This is often an effective way to release the pain. Above all, you must forgive yourself if you are burdened by self-blame.

From time to time, the new parents may need to remind themselves that though cesarean surgery is an unfortunate event, it is after all still an occasion to celebrate. A child is born.

Notes

CHAPTER ONE

1. *Am. J. Pub. Health,* Vol. 77, No. 2, p. 241, Feb 1987.
2. Ibid.
3. Porreco, Richard, "High Cesarean Section Rate: A New Perspective," *Obstetrics & Gynecology,* Vol. 65, No. 3 (March 1985), p. 307.
4. Haverkamp, A., et al., "The Evaluation of Continuous Fetal Heart Rate Monitoring in High-Risk Pregnancy," *Am. J. Ob. Gyn.,* Vol. 125, No. 3 (June 1976), p. 310.
5. Porreco, R., "High Cesarean Section Rate: A New Perspective," *Obstetrics & Gynecology,* Vol. 65, No. 3 (March 1985), p. 307.
6. Gilstrap, L., J. Hauth, and S. Toussaint, "Cesarean Section: Changing Incidence and Indications," *Obstetrics & Gynecology,* Vol. 63, No. 2 (February 1984).
7. O'Driscoll, K., and M. Foley, "Correlation of Decrease in Perinatal Mortality and Increase in Cesarean Section Rates," *Obstetrics & Gynecology,* Vol. 61, No. 1 (1983).
8. National Institutes of Health, *Cesarean Childbirth*, publication no. 82–2067, Bethesda, MD (October 1981), p. 4.

9. Williams, R., and P. Chen, "Controlling the Rise in Cesarean Section Rates by the Dissemination of Information from Vital Records," *Am. J. Public Health,* Vol. 73, pp. 863–867 (1983).
10. Eggers, Peggy, "Born in Love," *C/Sec Newsletter*, Vol. 12, No. 3 (1986), p. 1.
11. Minkoff, H., and R. Schwarz, "The Rising Cesarean Section Rate: Can It Safely Be Reversed?" *Obstetrics & Gynecology,* Vol. 56, No. 2 (August 1980), p. 140.
12. National Institutes of Health, op. cit., p. 16.
13. Marut, J., and R. Mercer, "Comparison of Primiparas' Perception of Vaginal and Cesarean Births," *Nursing Research,* Vol. 28, No. 5 (September/October 1979).
14. Gleicher, N., "Cesarean Section Rates in the United States," *JAMA,* Vol. 252, No. 23 (December 21, 1984).
15. Marut and Mercer, op. cit., p. 265.
16. Royall, Nicki, *You Don't Need to Have a Repeat Cesarean* (New York: Frederick Fells Publishers, Inc., 1983), p. 2.
17. May, K., and D. Sollid, "Unanticipated Cesarean Birth from the Father's Perspective," *Birth,* Vol. 11:2 (Summer 1984).
18. Gleicher, N., "Cesarean Section Rates in the United States," *JAMA,* Vol. 252, No. 23 (December 21, 1984).
19. Royall, op. cit., pp. 104, 182.
20. Shearer, M., "Complications of Cesarean to Mother and Infant," *Birth & Family J.*, 4 (Fall 1977), No. 3.
21. Schreiner, R., et al., "Respiratory Distress Following Elective Repeat Cesarean Section," *Am. J. Ob. Gyn.*, Vol. 143, No. 6 (July 15, 1982).
22. Goldenberg, R., and K. Nelson, "Iatrogenic Respiratory Distress Syndrome: Analysis of Obstetric Events Preceding Delivery of Infants Who Develop Respiratory Distress Syndrome," *Am. J. Ob. Gyn.*, Vol. 123, p. 617 (1975).
23. Hack, M., Fanaroff, A., Klaus, M. et al., "Neonatal Respiratory Distress Following Elective Delivery: A Preventable Disease?" *Am. J. Ob. Gyn.*, Vol. 126, p. 43 (1976).
24. Schreiner, op. cit.
25. Lagercrantz, H., and T. Slotkin, "The 'Stress' of Being Born," April, 1986, Scientific American, pp. 100–107.
26. Ibid.

CHAPTER TWO

1. *Boston Globe* (October 21, 1984).
2. Kibrick, S., "Herpes Simplex Infection at Term," *JAMA*, Vol. 243, No. 2 (January 11, 1980), p. 157.
3. *C/Sec Newsletter*, Vol. 11, No. 4. (October 1985), p. 1.
4. *Am. J. Public Health*, Vol. 75, No. 2 (February 1985), p. 190.
5. National Institutes of Health, *Cesarean Childbirth*, publication no. 82–2067, Bethesda, MD (October 1981), p. 12.
6. Ibid.,
7. Hannah, W., "X-Ray Pelvimetry—A Critical Appraisal," *Am. J. Ob. Gyn.* (February 1, 1963), Vol. 91, No. 3.
8. Russell, J., "Moulding of the Pelvic Outlet," *J. Ob. Gyn. Brit. Cwlth.*, Vol. 76, pp. 817–20 (September 1969).
9. Barton, J., et al., "The Efficacy of X-Ray Pelvimetry," *Am. J. Ob. Gyn.*, Vol. 143, p. 304–11 (1982).
10. Quilligan, E., "Making Inroads Against the C-Section Rate," *Contemporary Ob/Gyn* (January 1983).
11. National Institutes of Health, op. cit., p. 342.
12. Klein, L., "Cesarean Birth and Trial of Labor," *The Female Patient*, Vol. 9 (September 1984).
13. Lederman, R., et al., "Anxiety and Epinephrine in Multiparous Women in Labor: Relationship to Duration of Labor and Fetal Heart Rate Pattern," *Am. J. Ob. Gyn.*, 153:870–7 (1985).
14. Notzon, F. C., Placck, P. J., and Tuffel, S. M., "Comparisons of National Cesarean-section Rates," N. Eng. J. of Med. 1987, 316:386–9.
15. National Institutes of Health, op. cit., p. 13.
16. Ibid., p. 14.
17. "Indications for Cesarean Section: Final Statement of the Panel of the National Consensus Conference on Aspects of Cesarean Birth," *CMAJ*, Vol. 134 (June 15, 1986), p. 1350.
18. Ibid.
19. Huchcroft, S., M. Wearing, and C. Buck, "Late Results of Cesarean and Vaginal Delivery in Cases of Breech Presentation," *CMAJ*, Vol. 125 (October 1, 1981), p. 729.
20. Mann, L., and J. Gallant, "Modern Management of the

Breech Delivery," *Am. J. Ob. Gyn.*, Vol. 134, p. 611–614 (1979).

21. Chervenak, F., et al., "Is Routine Cesarean Section Necessary for Vertex-Breech and Vertex-Transverse Twin Gestations?" *Am. J. Ob. Gyn.*, Vol. 148, No. 1 (January 1, 1984).
22. Karp, L., et al., "The Premature Breech: Trial of Labor or Cesarean Section?" *Obstetrics & Gynecology*, Vol. 53, No. 1 (January 1979).
23. DeSa Souza, J., "Postural Exercise Turns Fetus in Breech Position," *Ob. Gyn. News,* Vol. 12, No. 1 (January 1, 1977).
24. Quilligan, E., "Making Inroads against the C-Section Rate," *Contemporary Ob/Gyn* (January 1983).
25. Ranney, B., "The Gentle Art of External Cephalic Version," *Am. J. Ob. Gyn.*, Vol. 116, p. 239 (1973).
26. Garite, T., "External Cephalic Version," *C/Sec Newsletter*, Vol. 10, No. 1 (January 1984).
27. "Advances in Acupuncture and Acupuncture Anesthesia," People's Medical Clearing House, People's Republic of China, 1980; cited in Burstein, J., "Turning Breech Babies with Traditional Oriental Medicine," *C/Sec Newsletter*, Vol. 10, No. 2 (April 1984).
28. National Institutes of Health, op. cit., p. 391.

CHAPTER THREE

1. Notson, op. cit.
2. Caire, J., "Are Current Rates of Cesarean Justified?" *Southern Medical Journal*, Vol. 71, No. 5 (May 1978).
3. National Institutes of Health, *Antenatal Diagnosis*, publication no. 79–1973, Bethesda, MD, (April 1979).
4. Kelso, I., et al., "An Assessment of Continuous Fetal Heart Rate Monitoring in Labor," *Am. J. Ob. Gyn.*, Vol. 131, No. 5, pp. 526–532 (1978).
5. Caire, op. cit.
6. Shearer, M., "Fetal Monitoring: For Better or Worse?" *Compulsory Hospitalization*, Vol. 1, Stewart & Stewart, eds., (Marble Hill, MO: NAPSAC Publications, 1979), p. 126.

7. Ibid., p. 127.
8. Minkoff, H., and R. Schwarz, "The Rising Cesarean Section Rate: Can It Safely Be Reversed?" *Obstetrics & Gynecology,* Vol. 56, No. 2 (August 1980).
9. Haverkamp, A., et al., "The Evaluation of Continuous Fetal Heart Rate Monitoring in High-Risk Pregnancy," *Am. J. Ob. Gyn.*, Vol. 125, No. 3 (June 1, 1976).
10. Gassner, C., and W. Ledger, "The Relationship of Hospital-Acquired Maternal Infection to Invasive Intrapartum Monitoring Techniques," *Am. J. Ob. Gyn.*, Vol. 126, p. 33 (1976).
11. Haverkamp, A., "Does Anyone Need Fetal Monitors?" *Compulsory Hospitalization*, Vol. 1, Stewart & Stewart, eds. (Marble Hill, MO: NAPSAC Publications, 1979), p. 137.
12. Gilstrap, L., J. Hauth, and S. Toussaint, "Cesarean Section: Changing Incidence and Indications," *Obstetrics & Gynecology*, Vol. 63, No. 2 (February 1984).
13. Paul, R., J. Huey, and C. Yeager, "Clinical Fetal Monitoring: Its Effect on Cesarean Section Rate and Perinatal Mortality: Five-Year Trends," *Postgrad Med*, Vol. 61, p. 160 (1977).
14. Caire, op. cit.
15. Haverkamp, A., et al., "The Evaluation of Continuous Fetal Heart Rate Monitoring in High-Risk Pregnancy," p. 316.
16. Lagercrantz, H., and T. Slotkin, "The 'Stress' of Being Born," April, 1986, *Scientific American*, pp. 100–107.
17. Kubli, F., "Influence of Labor on Fetal Acid-Base Balance," *Clin. Ob. Gyn.*, Vol. 11, pp. 168–191 (1968).
18. Lumley, J., and C. Wood, "Transient Fetal Acidosis and Artificial Rupture of the Membranes," *Aust. NZ. J. Obstet Gynec.*, 11:221–225 (1971), cited in Lynaugh, K., "The Effects of Early Elective Amniotomy on the Length of Labor and the Condition of the Fetus," *Journal of Nurse-Midwifery*, Vol. 25, No. 4 (July/August 1980).
19. Friedman, E., and M. Sachtelben, "Amniotomy and the Course of Labor," *Ob. Gyn.*, 22:755–770 (1963).
20. Caldeyro-Barcia, R., et al., "Adverse Perinatal Effects of Early Amniotomy During Labor," *Modern Perinatal*

Medicine, L. Gluck, ed. (Chicago: Year Book Medical Publishers, 1974).

21. Schwarcz, R., et al., "Influence of Amniotomy and Maternal Position on Labor," *Gynecology & Obstetrics*, Caslelazo-Ayala et al., eds., (Amsterdam: *Excerpta Medica* 1977).
22. Haire, D., *The Cultural Warping of Childbirth*, (Milwaukee: ICEA, 1972).
23. Stewart, D., and L. Stewart, *The Childbirth Activists' Handbook*, (Marble Hill, MO: NAPSAC Publications, 1983), p. 67.
24. National Institutes of Health, *Cesarean Childbirth*, publication no. 82–2067, Bethesda, MD (October 1981), p. 482.
25. Jacobs, H., ed., *Obstetrical Malpractice*, Medical Quality Foundation (1979).
26. National Institutes of Health, op. cit., p. 479.
27. Gregg, S., "Family Wins $600,000 Settlement," *The Washington Post*, April 14, 1983.
28. Sandberg, E., in Graham, R., "Trial Labor Following Previous Cesarean Section," *Am. J. Ob. Gynec.*, Vol. 149, No. 1 (May 1, 1984), p. 42.
29. Goldfarb, M., "Who Receives Cesareans: Patient and Hospital Characteristics," National Center for Health Services Research, DHHS Publication no. 84–3345 (September 1984), p. 3.
30. National Institutes of Health, op. cit., p. 131.
31. Placek, P., Taffel, S., Moien, M., "Cesarean Section Delivery Rates: United States, 1981," *Am. J. Public Health*, 73:861–862 (1983).
32. National Institutes of Health, op. cit., p. 129.
33. *American Journal of Public Health*, Vol. 75, No. 2 (February 1985).
34. Gleicher, N., "Cesarean Section Rates in the United States," *JAMA*, Vol. 252, No. 23 (December 21, 1984).
35. Goldfarb, M., op. cit., p. 15.

CHAPTER FOUR

1. Stewart, D., and L. Stewart, *The Childbirth Activists' Handbook,* (Marble Hill, MO: NAPSAC Reproductions, 1983), p. 67.
2. Newton, N., *Maternal Emotions,* (New York: Paul B. Hoeber, 1982).
3. Jensen, M., Benson, R., Bobak, I., *Maternity Care: The Nurse and the Family,* 2nd edition (New York: C. V. Mosby Co., 1981).
4. Marut, J., "The Special Needs of the Cesarean Mother," *Am. J. Maternal-Child Nursing* (July/August 1978), p. 203.
5. Panuthos, C., "The Psychological Effects of Cesarean Deliveries," *Mothering*, (Winter 1983).
6. Cohen, N., and L. Estner, *Silent Knife*, (S. Hadley, MA: Bergin & Garvey, 1983).
7. Jones, IIC., *Mind Over Labor*, (New York: Viking/Penguin, 1987).
8. Goldfarb, M., "Who Receives Cesareans: Patient and Hospital Characteristics," National Center for Health Services Research, DHHS Publication no. 84–3345 (September 1984), p. 3.
9. Ibid., p. 15.
10. Haverkamp, A., "Does Anyone Need Fetal Monitors?" *Compulsory Hospitalization,* Vol. 1, Stewart & Stewart, eds. (Marble Hill, MO: NAPSAC Publications, 1979), p. 138.

CHAPTER FIVE

1. Liu, Y., "Position During Labor and Delivery: History and Perspective," *Journal of Nurse-Midwifery*, Vol. 24, No. 3 (May/June 1979).
2. Russell, J., "The Rationale of Primitive Delivery Positions," *Bri. J. Obstet. Gynaec.*, 89:712–15 (1982), cited in *C/Sec Newsletter*, Vol. 12, No. 2 (1986).
3. Hilbers, S., cited in Jones, C., *Mind Over Labor* (New York: Viking/Penguin, 1987), p. 12.
4. Ibid.
5. Newton, N., "The Effect of Fear and Disturbance on Labor," *in 21st Century Obstetrics Now!* Vol. 1, Stewart & Stewart,

eds. (Marble Hill, MO: NAPSAC, Inc., July 1977), pp. 63–71.
6. Ventre, F., cited in *C/Sec Newsletter*, Vol. 12, No. 2 (1986).

CHAPTER SIX

1. National Institutes of Health, *Cesarean Childbirth,* Publication no. 82–2067, Bethesda, MD (October 1981), p. 353.
2. Gleicher, N., "Cesarean Section Rates in the United States," *JAMA,* Vol. 252, No. 23 (December 21, 1984).
3. Craigin, E., *N.Y. J. Med.*, 104:1 (1916).
4. Meier, P., and R. Porreco, "Trial of Labor Following Cesarean Section: A Two-Year Experience," *Am. J. Ob. Gyn.*, Vol. 144, No. 6 (November 15, 1982), p. 675.
5. Minkoff, H., and R. Schwarz, "The Rising Cesarean Section Rate: Can It Safely Be Reversed?" *Obstetrics & Gynecology,* Vol. 56, No. 2 (August 1980), pp. 137–38.
6. National Institutes of Health, op. cit., ch. 11.
7. Pauerstein C., "Labor After Cesarean Section, From Precept to Practice," *J. Reprod. Med.*, 26:409 (1981), cited in P. Meier, and R. Porreco, "Trial of Labor Following Cesarean Section: A Two-Year Experience," *Am. J. Ob. Gyn.*, Vol. 144, No. 6 (November 15, 1982), p. 675.
8. Ibid., p. 676.
9. Ibid., pp. 675–76.
10. National Institutes of Health, op. cit., p. 43.
11. Porreco, R., and P. Meier, "Repeat Cesareans—Mostly Unnecessary," *Contemporary Ob/Gyn*, (September 1984), pp. 56–57.
12. National Institutes of Health, Ibid., p. 44.
13. Muller, P., Heiser, W., Graham, W., "Repeat Cesarean Section," *Am. J. Ob. Gyn.*, Vol. 81, p. 867 (1961).
14. Cohen, N., and L. Estner, *Silent Knife* (S. Hadley, MA: Bergin & Garvey, 1983), p. 83.
15. Meier, P., "Trial of Labor After Cesarean Section," paper presented at *Birth & Family J.* Conference, San Francisco, October 16–17, 1981. Cited in *Silent Knife*, Ibid., p. 95.
16. Shearer, E., "Education for Vaginal Birth After Cesarean," *Birth*, Vol. 9, p. 1 (Spring 1982).

17. Paul, R., et al., "Trial of Labor in the Patient with a Prior Cesarean Birth," *Am. J. Ob. Gyn.*, Vol. 151, No. 3 (February 1, 1985), p. 303.
18. Lavin, J., "Vaginal Delivery After Cesarean Birth: Frequently Asked Questions," *Clinics in Perinatology*, Vol. 10, No. 2 (June 1983), p. 443.
19. Shearer, B., and A. Cane, eds., *Frankly Speaking*, 3rd edition, (Framingham, MA: C/Sec, Inc., 1984).
20. Lavin, J., et al., "Vaginal Delivery in Patients with a Prior Cesarean Section," *Ob. Gyn.*, Vol. 59, pp. 135–148 (February 1982).
21. Douglas, R., et al., "Pregnancy and Labor Following Cesarean Section," *Am. J. Ob. Gyn.* Vol. 86, p. 961 (August 1963).
22. Morewood, C., et al., "Vaginal Delivery After Cesarean Section," *Obstetrics & Gynecology*, Vol. 42, No. 4 (October 1973).
23. Ibid.
24. Cohen and Estner, op. cit., p. 86.
25. Shearer, E., "Preventing Unnecessary Cesareans," C/Sec, Inc. (1982).
26. Am. J. Public Health, Vol. 77, No. 2, p. 241, Feb. 1987.
27. Cohen, R., "Letters to the Editor," *C/Sec Newsletter*, Vol. 10, No. 1 (January 1984).
28. Meier and Porreco, "Trial of Labor Following Cesarean Section: A Two-Year Experience," op. cit.
29. Cohen and Estner, op. cit., p. 89.
30. Lavin, J., et al., "Vaginal Delivery in Patients with a Prior Cesarean Section,"
31. Meier and Porreco, "Trial of Labor Following Cesarean Section: A Two-Year Experience," op. cit., p. 674.
32. Ibid., p. 677.
33. Gellman, E., et al., "Vaginal Delivery After Cesearean Section," *JAMA*, Vol. 249, No. 21 (June 3, 1983).
34. Meier and Porreco, "Trial of Labor Following Cesarean Section: A Two-Year Experience," op. cit., p. 672.
35. Porreco and Meier, "Repeat Cesareans—Mostly Unnecessary," op. cit., p. 56.

36. Ibid., p. 62.
37. Klein, L., "Cesarean Birth and Trial of Labor," *The Female Patient*, Vol. 9 (September 1984), p. 117.
38. Lavin, et al., op. cit., p. 145.
39. Porreco and Meier, "Repeat Cesareans—Mostly Unnecessary," op. cit., p. 56.
40. Consensus Conference Report: "Indications for Cesarean Section: Final Statement of the Panel of the National Consensus Conference on Aspects of Cesarean Birth," *CMAJ*, Vol. 134 (June 15, 1986).
41. Horenstein, J., and J. Phelan, "Previous Cesarean Section: The Risks and Benefits of Oxytocin Usage in a Trial of Labor," *Am. J. Ob. Gyn.*, Vol. 151, No. 5 (March 1, 1985).
42. Lavin, J., "Vaginal Delivery After Cesarean Birth: Frequently Asked Questions," *Clinics in Perinatology*, Vol. 10, No. 2 (June 1983), p. 449.
43. Meier and Porreco, "Trial of Labor Following Cesarean Section: A Two-Year Experience," op. cit., p. 676.
44. Paul, et al., op. cit., p. 299.
45. Porreco, R., and P. Meier, "Trial of Labor in Patients with Multiple Previous Cesarean Sections," *Journal of Reproductive Medicine*, Vol. 28, No. 11 (November 1983), p. 770.
46. Riva, H., and S. Teich, "Vaginal Delivery After Cesarean Section," *Am. J. Ob. Gyn.*, Vol. 81, p. 501 (1961).
47. Saldana, L., et al., "Management of Pregnancy After Cesarean Section," *Am. J. Ob. Gyn.*, Vol. 135, p. 555 (1979).
48. Porreco and Meier, "Repeat Cesareans—Mostly Unnecessary," op. cit., p. 56.
49. Lavin, J., et al., "Vaginal Delivery in Patients with a Prior Cesarean Section," *Obstetrics & Gynecology*, Vol. 59, No. 2 (February 1982), p. 146.

CHAPTER SEVEN

1. Cohen, M., and B. Carson, "Respiratory Morbidity Benefit of Awaiting Onset of Labor After Elective Cesarean Section," *Obstetrics & Gynecology*, Vol. 65: pp. 818–824 (1985).

2. Schreiner, R., et al., "Respiratory Distress Following Elective Repeat Cesarean Section," *Am. J. Ob. Gyn.*, Vol. 143, No. 6 (July 15, 1982), p. 692.
3. Lavin, J., et al., "Vaginal Delivery in Patients with a Prior Cesarean Section," *Obstetrics & Gynecology*, Vol. 59, No. 2 (February 1982), p. 147.
4. E. Snedemark, quoted in *The New York Times*, "Fathers Attending Cesarean Births," July 11, 1985, pp. C1–9.
5. Cronenwett, L., and L. Newmark, "Fathers' Responses to Childbirth," *Nursing Research*, 23:210–217 (May/June 1974).
6. Brazelton, T., *On Becoming a Father* (New York: Delacorte Press, 1981).
7. Marut, J., "The Special Needs of the Cesarean Mother," *Am. J. Maternal-Child Nursing* (July/August 1978), p. 206.
8. McClellan, M., and W. Cabianca, "Effects of Early Mother-Infant Contact Following Cesarean Birth," *Obstetrics & Gynecology*, Vol. 56, No. 1 (July 1980).
9. Royall, N., *You Don't Need to Have a Repeat Cesarean*, (New York: Frederick Fell Publishers, Inc., 1983), p. 129.
10. Gibson, K., "Our Cesarean Trauma: A Father's Reaction," *C/Sec Newsletter*, Vol. 10, No. 2 (April 1984).

Resources

SUPPORT AND INFORMATION

C/Sec, Inc.
22 Forest Road
Framingham, MA 01701
(617) 877-8266

C/Sec provides information on cesarean prevention and vaginal birth after cesarean, as well as support for cesarean families through telephone and person-to-person contact.

C/Sec also publishes an extremely informative and well-researched newsletter about issues relating to cesarean prevention and surgery. Membership is $15 yearly.

The Cesarean Prevention Movement (CPM)
P.O. Box 152, University Station
Syracuse, NY 13210
(315) 424-1942

CPM offers information and support on cesarean prevention,

vaginal birth after cesarean, and publishes an informative and highly interesting newsletter, *The Clarion.* Membership is $20 yearly, which includes the newsletter and chapter membership.

CPM has fifty-five chapters throughout the country. Write or call for the chapter nearest your home.

NAPSAC International, Inc. (The National Association of Parents and Professionals for Safe Alternatives in Childbirth)
P.O. Box 646
Marble Hill, MO 63764
(314) 238-2010

Helpful information on all aspects of pregnancy, safe alternatives in childbirth (both in and out of the hospital), vaginal birth after cesarean, breastfeeding, infant care, and child rearing. Publishes *Directory of Alternative Birth Services* listing caregivers, birth centers, family-centered hospitals, childbirth educators, breastfeeding counselors, and more. Publishes newsletter, *NAPSAC News.* Write for free brochure, membership information, and catalogue.

CHILDBEARING CENTERS

To find a childbearing center near your home, write or call the National Association of Childbearing Centers (NACC): RFD 1, Box 1, Perkiomenville, Pennsylvania, 18074, 215-234-8068 (Enclose a self-addressed stamped envelope).

BREASTFEEDING

La Leche League International
9616 Minneapolis Avenue
Franklin Park, IL 60131
(312) 455-7730

Provides information and support about nursing at no cost. Monthly meetings throughout the United States. Publishes many informative pamphlets (send for current catalogue) and a bimonthly newsletter, *New Beginnings,* sent to all members. Membership costs $20 yearly ($25 in Canada).

Check the telephone directory for a La Leche League leader near your home. If there is no listing, call the main number for a referral.

La Leche League maintains a twenty-four-hour hotline. For information, call the main number.

There are many other nursing mothers' groups throughout the country. Contact local childbirth education groups and maternity centers for names in your area.

HERPES

"Herpes and Pregnancy" (fact sheet)
The Herpes Resource Center
American Health Association
P.O. Box 100
Palo Alto, CA 94306
(415) 328-7710

"Herpes in Pregnancy" by Carla Reinke (four-page pamphlet)
Pennypress, Inc.
1100 23rd Avenue East
Seattle, WA 98112
(206) 325-1419

"Herpes" (nine-page pamphlet)
Council for Cesarean Awareness
5520 S.W. 92nd Avenue
Miami, FL 33165
(305) 666-7090

Suggested Reading

CHILDBIRTH PREPARATION AND LABOR

Bean, Constance A., *Methods of Childbirth*. New York: Doubleday & Co., 1972.

Jones, Carl, *Sharing Birth: A Father's Guide to Giving Support During Labor.* New York: William Morrow & Co., 1985.

Jones, Carl, Henci Goer, and Penny Simkin, "The Labor Support Guide—For Fathers, Family and Friends" (Pamphlet—order directly from Pennypress, Inc., 1100 23rd Avenue East, Seattle, WA 98112 [$1.00]).

Korte, Diana, and Roberta Skaer, *A Good Birth, A Safe Birth.* New York: Bantam 1984.

CESAREAN

Cohen, Nancy, and Lois Estner, *Silent Knife.* S. Hadley, MA: Bergin & Garvey, 1983.

Donovan, Bonnie, *The Cesarean Birth Experience.* Boston: Beacon Press, 1978.

Cesarean Childbirth. The National Institute of Health Consensus Report, available by writing: The National Institute of Child Health and Human Development, 9000 Rockville Pike, Bldg. 31, Room 2A32, Bethesda, MD 20892; or call (301) 496-5133.

GRIEVING

Friedman, Rochelle, and Bonnie Gradstein, *Surviving Pregnancy Loss.* Boston: Little, Brown, 1982.

Panuthos, Claudia, *Ended Beginnings: Healing Childbearing Losses.* S. Hadley, MA: Bergin & Garvey, 1984.

MISCELLANEOUS

Elkins, Valmai, *The Rights of the Pregnant Parent.* New York: Schocken Books, 1976.

Stewart, David, *The Five Standards of Safe Childbearing.* Marble Hill, MO: NAPSAC, Inc., 1981.

Stewart, David, and Lee Stewart, eds., *21st Century Obstetrics Now!* (2 volumes), Marble Hill, MO: NAPSAC, Inc., 1977.

Stewart, David, and Lee Stewart, eds., *Compulsory Hospitalization: Freedom of Choice in Childbirth?* (2 volumes), Marble Hill, MO: NAPSAC, Inc., 1979.

FATHERS

Bittman, Sam, and Sue R. Zalk, *Expectant Fathers.* New York: Ballantine, 1981.

Greenberg, Martin, *The Birth of a Father.* New York: Continuum, 1985.

THE POSTPARTUM PERIOD

Jones, Carl, *After the Baby Is Born.* New York: Dodd, Mead & Co., 1986.

Jones, Carl, and Larry Snydal, *The New Father's Survival Guide.* New York: Franklin Watts, 1987.

Fienup-Riordan, Ann, *Shape Up With Baby.* Seattle: Pennypress, Inc., 1980.

Whiteford, Barbara, and Margie Polden, *The Postnatal Exercise Book.* New York: Pantheon, 1984.

BREASTFEEDING

Eiger, Marvin, and Sally Olds, *The Complete Book of Breastfeeding.* New York: Bantam, 1973.

La Leche League International, *The Womanly Art of Breastfeeding.* New York: New American Library, 1958.

Pryor, Karen, *Nursing Your Baby.* New York: Pocket Books, 1973.

All of the above titles are available from:

Birth & Life Bookstore
P.O. Box 70625
Seattle, WA 98107
(206) 789-4444

Phone orders with Master Card, Visa, or UPS COD accepted.

Birth & Life Bookstore also publishes *Imprints,* a quarterly review of current works about childbearing and parenthood. Mailed free.

NAPSAC Bookstore
P.O. Box 646
Marble Hill, MO 63764
(314) 238-2010

Tapes for Mental Imagery

Great Expectations—The Joy of Pregnancy and Birthing By Emmett Miller, M.D. One side is a guide through pregnancy from conception to delivery; the other is designed to increase confidence and promote greater relaxation and enjoyment during birth. (Available for $10.95 from Source, P.O. Box W, Stanford, CA 94305 or call 415-328-7171, or 1-800-TAPES in states outside of California.)

The Child Within by Leni Schwartz, Ph.D. Six meditations for pregnant couples, to enhance the experience of pregnancy and develop a relationship with the child while it is still in the womb. (Available for $9.98 from Leni Schwartz, 325 Sanchez, Santa Fe, NM 87501.)

Relaxation and Visualization in Preparation for Childbirth by June Whitson and Roxanne Cummings. Relaxation and imagery exercises accompanied by music. (Available for $10.95 from June Whitson, Box 95, La Honda, CA 94020.)

Welcoming Your Creation Within by Rose Heman, R.N.C.P. The first side contains suggestions for communicating with and expressing your love for your baby before it is born. The second is a birth visualization directed at overcoming fears and negative beliefs while creating a positive, relaxed attitude for a fulfilling and loving birth experience. (Available for $12.95 from Rose Heman, R.N.C.P., P.O. Box 8168, West Bloomfield, MI 48304.)

Index

C

D

E

F

M

N

O

P

Q

R

T

U

V

W

Y

Z